P9-DWJ-571

THE SOUTH BEACH DIET

GOOD FATS GOOD CARBS GUIDE

Arthur Agatston, M.D.

Author of the *New York Times* Bestseller *The South Beach Diet*

RODALE

Special thanks to Marie Almon, R.D., our nutritionist, for her dedicated effort to this endeavor. Thanks also to Kathleen Hanuschak, R.D., and JoAnn Brader.

Printed in the United States of America
Rodale Inc. makes every effort to use acid-free a, recycled paper O.

Book design by Carol Angstadt

ISBN-10: 1–59486–198–6
ISBN-13: 978–1–59486–198–7

Distributed to the book trade by St. Martin's Press

10   9   paperback

We inspire and enable people to improve their lives and the world around them

For more of our products visit **rodalestore.com** or call 800-848-4735

CONTENTS

Foreword v

Your Road Map to South Beach Success 1

Frequently Asked Questions 22

How to Use the Food Guide 31

    Beans and Legumes 37

    Beverages 40

    Bread and Bread Products 45

    Breakfast Foods 48

    Candy and Candy Bars 55

    Cheese, Cheese Products, and Cheese Substitutes 57

    Condiments 61

    Crackers, Dips, and Snacks 62

    Desserts 65

    Eggs, Egg Dishes, and Egg Substitutes 70

    Fast Food 73

    Fats and Oils 78

    Fish and Shellfish 82

    Fruit and Fruit Juices 86

    Grains and Rice 90

    Gravies and Sauces 91

    Ice Cream and Frozen Desserts 92

    Meal Replacement Bars and Shakes .95

    Meats, Processed Meats, and Meat Substitutes 97

    Milk, Milk Products, and Milk Substitutes 105

    Nuts, Nut Butters, and Seeds 110

    Pasta and Pasta Dishes 112

    Pickles, Peppers, and Relish 114

    Pizza 114

    Poultry 116

    Salads and Salad Dressings 121

    Soups 125

    Sweeteners and Sweet Substitutes 127

    Vegetables 129

The South Beach Supermarket Cheat Sheet 133

Medley of Menu Makeovers 136

The South Beach Dining-Out Guide 138

Index 144

FOREWORD

A good diet is always, to some degree, a work in progress. This is true of the South Beach Diet for two very sound reasons.

First, scientists are always conducting more and better research, and as a result we're always learning new facts about how our bodies make use of the food we eat. Given the seriousness of obesity and poor nutrition today, it makes sense that researchers are trying hard to determine what we can do, as individuals and as a society, to maintain our health and our waistlines. We are always working to incorporate the most important new findings into the South Beach Diet. This program is built on a foundation of science, but no one has the time to review scientific literature on a daily basis. So in the end, it all comes down to the question each one of us asks ourselves several times a day: "What should I eat?"

Second, the South Beach Diet has now been adopted by millions of people all over the world. We get huge amounts of feedback every day through the diet's Web site, by mail, and by every other means imaginable. We're constantly talking with people who are doing their best to incorporate the diet into their lifestyles. All that discussion has made us wiser in the ways that people actually put the diet to use.

I mention all this to alert you to the fact that we have made several improvements to this guide.

The biggest change is in the way we present the information in the charts that make up the main text: We now give more detail than in previous editions. For all the foods listed, you will now find figures giving Total Carbohydrates, Total Sugar, Total Fat and Saturated Fat, and Fiber. And for each food, we offer a recommendation for each phase of the diet. A more detailed explanation of the new information can be found in "How to Use the Food Guide" on page 31.

In keeping with the research I mentioned above, we've also modified our views on certain foods like tomatoes, carrots, and low-fat dairy. Whether it's a fruit or a vegetable, a tomato tastes great and contains good nutrients, like lycopene, which may help prevent cancer. They are low in fructose and so their glycemic index number (one of the things we take into account when looking at foods) is low, too. These foods are fine to eat in all phases of the diet, even during Phase 1, the strictest phase.

Carrots are no longer banned in Phase 2. Early studies determined that this vegetable had a high glycemic index, which is why we discouraged dieters from eating it. But newer research has changed this view. Also, carrots aren't calorie dense, meaning that you'd have to eat a huge amount of them in order to raise your blood sugar.

Bananas also have benefited from research on the glycemic index and the glycemic load of foods. A medium-size banana has a low glycemic index and a moderate glycemic load, making it an acceptable fruit for Phase 2.

Calcium may help control body fat, and recent studies indicate that there is actually a lower risk of obesity among people who eat dairy products regularly. We advise everyone to stick with low-fat or even non-fat dairy products: 1% or fat-free milk; non-fat yogurt, low-fat or part-skim cheese. We strongly advise dieters to avoid butter, cream, and sour cream. (You should also be careful of what you replace the butter with—check the ingredients to make sure your vegetable-based spread doesn't contain partially hydrogenated oil.

We've also included more information about important food categories like fast foods and meal replacement bars. In a perfect world, fast food would never make an appearance in our diet; and we'd never be so rushed that we'd eat a packaged snack bar instead of real food. But we need all the help we can get to eat healthy while living a typical time-stressed contemporary lifestyle, so we've listed the information for those occasions when whole foods are simply not available.

Finally, as I've discovered via our South Beach Diet Web

site, dieters also have good questions that never presented themselves while I was writing the book. So this guide now contains a chapter of Frequently Asked Questions (and their answers) for each of the three phases.

Good luck with your efforts to lose weight and get healthy. I hope this guide helps you reach your goals.

YOUR ROAD MAP TO SOUTH BEACH SUCCESS

Welcome! I'm glad you've decided to try the South Beach Diet and have taken the first step toward a future filled with health and vitality.

The South Beach Diet can't be classified as a low-carb diet, a low-fat diet, or a high-protein diet. Its rules: Consume the right carbs and the right fats and learn to snack strategically. The South Beach Diet has been so widely successful because people lose weight without experiencing cravings or feeling deprived, or even feeling that they're *on* a diet. It allows you to enjoy "healthy" carbohydrates, rather than the kinds that contribute to weight gain, diabetes, and cardiovascular disease. You can eat a great variety of foods in a great variety of recipes. This prevents repetition and boredom, two obstacles to long-term success. Our goal is that the South

Beach Diet becomes a healthy lifestyle, not just a diet. The purpose of this guide is to help you to accomplish this with ease. Read on for more on the principles of the diet, how to use this Guide, and shopping and dining-out tips.

Good Fats, Bad Fats

Fat is an important part of a healthy diet. There's more and more evidence that many fats are good for us and actually reduce the risk of heart attack and stroke. They also help our sugar and insulin metabolism and therefore contribute to our goals of long-term weight loss and weight maintenance. And because good fats make foods taste better, they help us enjoy the journey to a healthier lifestyle. But not all fats are created equal—there are good fats and bad fats.

"Good" fats include monounsaturated fats, found in olive and canola oils, peanuts and other nuts, peanut butter, and avocados. Monounsaturated fats lower total and "bad" LDL cholesterol—which accumulates in and clogs artery walls—while maintaining levels of "good" HDL cholesterol, which carries cholesterol from artery walls and delivers it to the liver for disposal.

Omega-3 fatty acids—polyunsaturated fats found in cold-water fish, canola oil, flaxseeds, walnuts, almonds, and macadamia nuts—also count as good fat. Recent studies have shown that populations that eat more omega-3s, like Eskimos (whose diets are heavy on fish), have fewer serious health problems like heart disease and diabetes. There is evidence that omega-3 oils helps prevent or treat depression, arthritis, asthma, and colitis and help prevent cardiovascular deaths. You'll eat both monounsaturated fats and omega-3s in abundance in all three phases of the Diet.

"Bad fats" include saturated fats—the heart-clogging kind found in butter, fatty red meats, and full-fat dairy products.

"Very bad fats" are the manmade trans fats. Trans fats, which are created when hydrogen gas reacts with oil, are found in many packaged foods, including margarine, cookies, cakes, cake icings, doughnuts, and potato chips. Trans fats are worse than saturated fats; they are bad for our blood vessels, nervous systems, and waistlines.

As this Guide went to press, the Food and Drug Administration (FDA) ruled that by 2006, food manufacturers must list the amount of trans fats in their products on the label. (The natural trans fats in meat and milk, which act very differently in the body than the manmade kind, will not require labeling.) Until then, here are a few ways to reduce your intake of trans fats and saturated fats, South Beach style.

Go natural: Limit margarine, packaged foods, and fast food, which tend to contain high amounts of saturated and trans fats. **Make over your cooking methods:** Bake, broil, or grill rather than fry. **Lose the skin:** Remove the skin from chicken or turkey before you eat it. **Ditch the butter:** Cook with canola or olive oil instead of butter, margarine, or lard. **Slim down your dairy:** Switch from whole milk to fat-free or 1% milk.

Good Carbs, Bad Carbs

Carbohydrates, foods that contain simple sugars (short chains of sugar molecules) or starches (long chains of sugar

(continued on page 8)

The Trans-Fat Hot List

You've probably heard a lot in the news lately about trans fats—a particularly nasty type of fat that can wreak havoc on your health. Food manufacturers have not been required to list this type of fat on their food labels in the past, but because of new government regulations, manufacturers will be required to list the amount of trans fats in their products by 2006. Until then, here is what you need to know to identify trans fats present in foods.

Look for the words "hydrogenated" or "partially hydrogenated" oil on the list of ingredients. If it is listed as the first, second, or third ingredient, the food has a lot trans fats in it. The common names for trans fats to look for on food labels include partially hydrogenated soybean oil, partially hydrogenated corn oil, partially hydrogenated soybean and/or cottonseed oil, partially hydrogenated palm kernel oil, partially hydrogenated coconut oil, and partially hydrogenated vegetable oil shortening.

You can also refer to this "Hot List" of foods that are known to harbor trans fats. To keep your weight loss on track, and to maintain good health, it's best to avoid these foods as much as possible. There are plenty of great-tasting, healthier alternatives you can have instead—just check the food chart in this book!

BREADS AND BREAD PRODUCTS

Biscuits, made from mix

Biscuits or rolls, made from refrigerated dough

Coating mixes for fish, meat, or poultry

Stuffing mixes

Taco shells

White and wheat flour breads (some types)

BREAKFAST FOODS

Most commercial bakery items, such as:

Cinnamon buns

Danish

Doughnuts

Muffins

Pastries or bakery items with icing or frosting

Sweet rolls

Toaster tarts or strudel, plain or iced

CANDY

Most commercial confectionary, such as:

Caramels

Chocolate

Fruit chews

Hard candies with a creamy texture (some types)

Seasonal candy

Taffy-like candy

DESSERTS

Most commercially prepared items, such as:

Cake sprinkles, decorettes, or baking chips

Cakes and cake mixes

Cakes or cupcakes prepared with icing or frosting

Ice cream cakes

Pie crusts, such as traditional, graham cracker, and cookie crumb, and some pie fillings, such as chocolate

Pound cake and fat-free pound cake

Ready-to-spread frostings

(continued)

DESSERTS (CONT.)

Refrigerated cookie dough

Refrigerated cookie kits with icing

DIPS AND SNACKS

Bean dips (some types)

Cheese and pretzel snack kits

Cheese and cracker snack kits (some types)

Cheese puffs

Chocolate- or yogurt-covered snacks (most types)

Cookie snack kits

Cookies, most types such as chocolate chip and vanilla wafers

Corn chips

Crackers, including cheese-filled sandwich-type, cream-filled sandwich-type, saltine-type, snack crackers and some types of wheat crackers

Nacho cheese dips

Popcorn packaged for the microwave

Potato chips and potato sticks

Pretzels filled with imitation cheese

Pudding snacks, prepared

Tortilla chips (some types)

Weight-loss snack bars (some types)

FAST FOODS

Breakfasts with biscuit topping, made from biscuit mixes

Biscuits served with fast-food dinners

French fries

Fried apples or fast-food fruit pies

Fried chicken

Fried fish sandwiches

Mixed meals from a box that contain buttermilk biscuit topping, cornbread topping, dumplings, or pouched seasoning mix

Most deep-fried fast foods

FATS AND OILS

Light spreads (some types)

Margarine, hard stick and regular tub types

Vegetable shortening, regular and butter-flavored

FROZEN FOODS

Breaded fish sticks

Entrées (some types)

French fries

Fruit pies and pie crusts

Pancakes and French toast

Pastries, heat-and-eat or pastries with icing

Pizza and pizza crusts

Pot pies

Waffles and waffle sticks

MILK AND MILK PRODUCTS

International and instant latte coffees (some types)

Refrigerated fat-free nondairy creamers

Refrigerated nondairy creamers (some types)

Whipped toppings

SALADS AND SALAD DRESSINGS

Commercially prepared salad dressings (some types)

SOUPS AND STEWS

Bouillon cubes (some types)

Boxed onion soup and dip mix

Ramen noodle and soup cups (some types)

molecules), have been blamed for our epidemic of obesity and diabetes. This is only partially true, because there are both good and bad carbohydrates. The good carbs contain the important vitamins, minerals, and other nutrients that are essential to our health and that help prevent heart disease and cancer. The bad carbs, which have been consumed by Americans in unprecedented quantities (largely in an attempt to avoids fats), are the ones that have resulted in the fattening of America. Bad carbs are refined carbs, the ones where digestion has begun in factories instead of in our stomachs. The good carbs are the ones humans were designed to consume—the unrefined ones that have contributed to our health since we began eating! Unrefined carbohydrates are found in whole, natural foods, such as whole grains, legumes, rice, and starchy vegetables. They're also called complex carbohydrates, so named for their molecular structure. Besides being packed with fiber, vitamins, and minerals, good carbs take longer to digest—a good thing, as you'll soon see.

Refined carbohydrates, on the other hand, are found in packaged, processed foods, such as store-bought baked goods, crackers, pasta, and white bread.

Refined carbohydrates are made with white flour and contain little or no fiber. In fact, many products made with white flour are advertised as fortified with vitamins and minerals, because the process of turning grain into white flour strips away its fiber and nutrients. One of our South Beach Diet rules is to avoid foods labeled as "fortified." Current evidence is that fortification with vitamins does not recreate the benefits of the natural vitamins that have been removed.

Despite the fact that good carbs are a critical part of a healthy diet, the typical American diet is filled with the bad kinds. And when we're overweight as a result of a diet laden with bad carbs, our bodies' ability to process *all* carbohydrates goes awry. To understand why, you need to understand the role of the hormone insulin.

Insulin, Fat, and "Fast Sugar"

All foods, even natural foods like fruits and beans, contain naturally occurring sugar in some form. But there's a critical difference among these sugars: The body digests and absorbs them at different speeds.

When sugars from food enter the bloodstream, the pancreas produces insulin. It's insulin's job to move sugars out of the blood and into the cells, where they're either used or stored for future use. Insulin is the key that "unlocks" our cells and lets sugars in.

How much insulin is required to do that job depends on the foods we eat. Foods that are broken down and absorbed into the bloodstream quickly require a lot of insulin. Those that are metabolized and enter the blood more slowly require a gradual release of insulin.

In a nutshell, the quicker sugar floods the bloodstream, the quicker insulin rises. This is bad, both for your weight and for your general health.

Here's why: When glucose is absorbed slowly, the rise in

(continued on page 12)

Beyond Weight Loss: The South Beach Diet Benefits Your Health, Too

Has your doctor has told you that you must lose weight to stave off heart disease or diabetes? Then the South Beach Diet may be the one for you.

Why? Because the Diet that's helping millions across the nation shed their extra pounds *didn't start out as a weight-loss diet at all.* I created the Diet to help my patients lower their levels of cholesterol and triglycerides and to lower their risk of pre-diabetes (the condition that precedes full-blown type 2 diabetes and that has been linked to risk of heart attack and stroke).

And it's been proven to do just that.

To give just one example, one of my male patients in his midfifties had high blood pressure, high cholesterol, high triglycerides, and narrowing in his coronary arteries. His previous doctor had prescribed the usual medications. But once on the Diet, his cardiac profile quickly improved. His triglycerides, which had been over 400, fell below 100—a normal level—after just a month. He also lost 30 pounds, which he's kept off, and no longer takes all those heart medications.

The results of the Diet have also been measured in a scientific setting. My colleagues and I conducted a study pitting the Diet against the strict "step 2" American Heart Association diet. They randomized 40 overweight volunteers to either of the diets, meaning that half went on the Heart Association program and half got the South Beach Diet. None of the subjects knew where their diet had come from.

After 12 weeks, five patients on the Heart Association diet had given up, compared with one on the South Beach plan. The South Beach patients also showed a greater decrease in waist-to-hip ratio, suggesting a true decrease in cardiac risk. Triglycerides dramatically decreased for the South Beach dieters, and their good-to-bad cholesterol ratio improved more than that of the Heart Association group. Finally, the South Beach dieters experienced a mean weight loss of 13.6 pounds, almost double the 7.5 pounds lost by the Heart Association group.

blood sugar is gradual—and so is its fall, once insulin begins to work. A slow decline in blood sugar means fewer cravings later.

But when blood sugar rises quickly, the pancreas pumps out a correspondingly high level of insulin. The result? Blood sugar drops so low that it triggers new cravings. Often, we satisfy cravings by overeating (typically bad carbs like chips and candy bars), which leads to weight gain. Worse, the excess weight caused by overeating can lead to insulin resistance, the precursor to full-blown type 2 diabetes. In insulin resistance, cells ignore insulin's signal to accept glucose from the blood. As a result, the pancreas must crank out huge amounts of insulin until eventually the exhausted organ wears out.

Those of us who have grown protruding bellies while our arms and legs stay relatively thin are likely to have the syndrome of insulin resistance or "pre-diabetes." This occurs commonly in people with a family history of diabetes. Another sign of this syndrome is the occurrence of fatigue, weakness, headaches, irritability, shakiness, and cravings in the late morning or late afternoon. These are signs of exaggerated falls in blood sugar levels. The consumption of refined carbohydrates has unmasked this syndrome in approximately 25 percent of Americans and in the great majority of those of us who are overweight.

While eating the South Beach way will result in weight loss, it will also correct the way your body reacts to the very foods that made you heavy. It increases your body's sensitivity to insulin, thereby decreasing the swings in blood sugar that cause us to be hungry again, too soon after we finish a meal.

This metabolic transformation occurs in three phases. The

purpose of Phase 1 is to eradicate your cravings. You will accomplish this by eliminating all starches including all breads, potatoes, and rice. You will also eliminate all sugars, including all fruits and alcoholic beverages. You will enjoy strategic snacking, eating healthy snacks like nuts or low-fat cheese before your blood sugar dips too low in the late morning afternoon and/or evening. It takes much fewer calories to prevent those afternoon cravings than it does to satisfy those cravings once they hit. In Phase 1, nutrient rich vegetables and healthy salads are encouraged. You can expect to lose between 7 and 13 pounds during Phase 1.

In Phase 2, you'll gradually add back good carbohydrates, such as whole fruits and whole grains. Here's the principle for adding more carbs back safely: Do it gradually and attentively. The goal is to eat more carbs again while continuing to lose weight. If you add an apple and a slice of bread a day and you're still dropping pounds, that's great. If you try having an apple, two slices of bread, and a banana daily and notice that your weight loss has stalled, you've gone too far. It's time to cut back, or try some different carbs and monitor the results. You can enjoy a glass of red or white wine with a meal; drinking wine with a meal actually helps slow digestion. In this phase, weight loss is about 1 to 2 pounds per week. You learn which carbs you can enjoy without the return of cravings.

Once you have reached your weight loss goal, it is time for Phase 3, the maintenance phase. There are no absolute restrictions here, but you have learned the "pecking order" of the important food groups. You have learned to choose brown rice instead of white rice, sweet potatoes instead of white potatoes, and pita bread rather than white bread. This is where the South Beach Diet becomes a lifestyle. (For an idea of which foods to avoid and which foods to enjoy on the South Beach Diet, see the lists on the next pages.)

In the next section, you'll be introduced to a system that can help you limit foods that cause unhealthy, fat-producing spikes and dips in blood sugar and insulin and choose those that keep blood sugar steady, making it easier to lose weight and keep it off.

Introducing the Glycemic Index

The glycemic index (GI) is a system that ranks foods by how fast and how high they cause blood sugar to rise after eating a particular food. The GI of any particular food is always compared to a standard reference food, which is either one slice of white bread or a small amount of glucose, both of which have a numerical value of 100. The higher the glycemic index, the greater the swings in blood sugar produced. So, in general, the lower the glycemic index, the better the food choice. For mixed meals, the total glycemic index is approximately the average of the indices of the individual foods.

Generally speaking, you can think of GI in 3 ranges: "low" (55 and below), "medium" (56 to 69), and "high" (70 or above).

Foods with a low GI are converted to glucose more slowly, and so their sugars enter the bloodstream more slowly. Foods with a medium or high GI, which are converted to glucose more quickly, release their sugars into the blood-stream more rapidly. This results in a swifter rise in insulin.

Unrefined carbs often fall lower on the GI scale because they're rich in fiber, which takes longer to digest and so results in a slow, gradual rise in blood sugar.

How about refined, bad carbs? Not surprisingly, their processed sugars enter the bloodstream quickly. This quick conversion makes blood sugar and insulin rise and fall quickly—definitely not so good.

On the South Beach Diet, you'll tend to eat foods that fall lower on the GI, prepared or eaten in ways that allow your body to digest and absorb them more slowly. After Phase 1, the strictest phase of the Diet, you'll reintroduce good carbohydrates with a higher GI.

While the GI is an astounding breakthrough in our understanding of how carbohydrates affect our metabolism, there are a few important things you need to know to use the system successfully. First, the GI doesn't account for portion size. The solution: the concept of the glycemic load (GL), which takes into account a food's GI (the quality of carbohydrate) as well as the amount (the quantity of carbohydrate) per serving. It also represents the load, or stress, placed on the pancreas from the amount of carbohydrates consumed from a particular food or meal.

For this Guide, our evaluation of each food choice is based on the glycemic index, glycemic load, and on other factors as well. We don't include a dedicated column with a GI number for each entry because that information is not available for all of the 1,200 foods that are listed in these pages.

(continued on page 22)

Phase 1

The following is a list of foods that you can feel free to enjoy (as well as foods you'll need to avoid) when you begin Phase 1 of the South Beach Diet. These lists will help you stay on track and avoid carbohydrates that may crop up in foods where you don't expect them.

Foods to Enjoy

BEEF
Lean cuts, such as:
Sirloin (including ground)
Tenderloin
Top round

DAIRY
1% or fat-free milk
Plain fat-free yogurt
Low-fat plain soy milk (4 g of fat or less per serving)
1% or fat-free buttermilk

POULTRY (SKINLESS)
Cornish hen
Turkey bacon (2 slices per day)
Turkey and chicken breast

SEAFOOD
All types of fish and shellfish

PORK
Boiled ham
Canadian bacon
Tenderloin

VEAL
Chop
Cutlet, leg
Top round

LUNCHMEAT
Fat-free or low-fat only

CHEESE (REDUCED FAT)
American
Cheddar
Cottage cheese, 1%, 2%, or fat-free
Cream cheese substitute, dairy-free

Feta
Mozzarella
Parmesan
Provolone
Ricotta
String

NUTS
Almonds, 15
Cashews, 15
Macadamias, 8
Peanut butter, 2 tbsps
Peanuts, 20 small
Pistachios, 30

EGGS
Whole eggs are not limited unless otherwise directed by your doctor. Use egg whites and egg substitute as desired.

TOFU
Use soft, low-fat, or lite varieties

VEGETABLES AND LEGUMES
Artichokes
Asparagus
Beans
Broccoli
Cabbage
Cauliflower
Celery
Collard greens
Cucumbers
Eggplant
Lettuce (all varieties)
Mushrooms (all varieties)
Snow peas
Spinach
Sprouts, alfalfa
Tomatoes
Turnips
Water chestnuts
Zucchini

FATS
Oil, canola
Oil, olive

SPICES AND SEASONINGS
All spices that contain no added sugar
Broth
Extracts (almond, vanilla, or others)
Horseradish sauce
I Can't Believe It's Not Butter! spray
Pepper (black, cayenne, red, white)

(continued)

Foods to Enjoy (cont.)

**SWEET TREATS
(LIMIT TO 75 CALORIES
PER DAY)**
Candies, hard, sugar-free
Chocolate powder, no sugar added
Cocoa powder, baking type
Fudge pops, no sugar added
Gelatin, sugar-free
Gum, sugar-free
Popsicles, sugar-free
Sugar substitute

Foods to Avoid

BEEF
Brisket
Liver
Other fatty cuts
Rib steaks

POULTRY
Chicken, wings and legs
Duck
Goose
Poultry products, processed

PORK
Honey-baked ham

VEAL
Breast

CHEESE
Brie
Edam
Non reduced-fat

VEGETABLES

Beets

Corn

Potatoes, sweet

Potatoes, white

Yams

FRUIT

Avoid all fruits and fruit juices in Phase 1, including:

Apples

Apricots

Berries

Cantaloupe

Grapefruit

Peaches

Pears

STARCHES AND CARBS

Avoid all starchy food in Phase 1, including:

Bread, all types

Cereal

Matzo

Oatmeal

Pasta, all types

Pastry and baked goods, all types

Rice, all types

DAIRY

Avoid the following dairy in Phase 1:

Ice cream

Milk, whole or 2%

Soy milk, whole

Yogurt, cup-style and frozen

MISCELLANEOUS

Alcohol of any kind, including beer and wine

Phase 2

As with Phase 1, Phase 2 also has recommendations for which foods to eat. The first list tells you which foods to reintroduce into your diet. The second list includes foods that you'd best eat only rarely—any more than that could affect your blood glucose levels and derail your weight-loss efforts as well.

Foods You Can Reintroduce to Your Diet

VEGETABLES/LEGUMES
Barley
Beans, pinto
Black-eyed peas
Carrots

STARCHES (LIMIT)
Bagels, small, whole grain
Bread
    multigrain
    oat and bran
    rye
    whole wheat
Cereal
    Fiber One
    Kellogg's Extra-Fiber All-Bran
    Oatmeal (not instant)
    Other high-fiber
    Uncle Sam

Muffins, bran, sugar-free (no raisins)
Pasta, whole wheat
Peas, green
Pita
    stone-ground
    whole wheat
Popcorn
Potato, small, sweet
Rice
    brown
    wild

FRUIT
Apples
Apricots, dried or fresh
Bananas (medium)
Blueberries
Cantaloupe

Cherries
Grapefruit
Grapes
Kiwi
Mangoes
Oranges
Peaches
Pears
Plums
Strawberries

DAIRY
Artifically sweetened nonfat
flavored yogurt, 4 oz cup per
day

MISCELLANEOUS
Chocolate (sparingly)
   bittersweet
   semisweet
Pudding, fat-free, sugar-free
Wine, red or white

Foods to Avoid or Eat Rarely

VEGETABLES
Beets
Corn
Potatoes, white

STARCHES AND BREADS
Bagel, refined wheat
Bread
  refined wheat
  white
Cookies
Cornflakes
Matzo
Pasta, white flour
Rice cakes
Rice, white
Rolls, dinner

FRUIT
Canned fruit, juice-packed
Fruit juice
Pineapple
Raisins
Watermelon

MISCELLANEOUS
Honey
Ice cream
Jam

FREQUENTLY ASKED QUESTIONS

PHASE 1

I don't like eggs. What else can I have for breakfast?

Eggs are recommended in the South Beach Diet because they are a good source of protein, but there are many other healthy substitutes. Since you don't like eggs, you can enjoy tofu, Canadian bacon, fat-free or low-fat cheese, plain yogurt, peanut butter, or the chicken, fish, or beef from last night's dinner—all foods high in protein. For more ideas, check out the "What to Eat—Phase 1" section of this book on page 16. Experiment with new ingredients and recipes until you find meals that work for you.

How many servings of nuts can I have?

Nuts contain heart-healthy, unsaturated fat and make a great South Beach Diet snack. However, while the South Beach Diet doesn't require you to count calories, even healthy foods can be diet busters if you overindulge. For this reason, we limit nuts to one serving daily. The serving size varies, depending on the type of nut (see guidelines below). To avoid overdoing it, measure out your snack and put the rest away.

Almonds	15 (dry roasted recommended)
Brazil nuts	4
Cashews	15 (dry roasted recommended)
Pecans	15 (dry roasted recommended)
Macadamia	8 (dry roasted recommended)
Peanut butter	2 tablespoons (natural recommended)
Peanuts	20 small (may use dry roasted or boiled)
Pine nuts (pignolia)	1 ounce
Pistachios	30 (dry roasted recommended)
Walnuts	15 (dry roasted recommended)

In place of nuts, you may use:

Flaxseed	3 tablespoons
Sunflower or pumpkin seeds	up to 1 ounce

What else can I drink besides water and vegetable juice?

Any diet, decaffeinated, sugar-free sodas and drinks are allowed on Phase 1. Be sure to check out the powdered drink mixes offered in your local grocery—there's an increasing variety of flavors like ruby red grapefruit, orange, iced tea, and pink lemonade.

In addition, you can enjoy 1 percent or fat-free milk and low-fat, plain soy milk (with 4 grams of fat or less per serving).

You can also drink caffeinated coffee or diet sodas with caffeine added—just try to limit your intake to 1 or 2 cups per day. Caffeine stimulates the pancreas to produce insulin, a hormone that regulates blood sugar. When too much insulin is released at once, it can result in cravings. However, 1 or 2 cups of coffee or caffeinated soda per day won't have much of an effect on insulin levels—so no need to completely deprive yourself!

I'm noticing "sugar alcohols" on labels I'm reading. What are they, and are they South Beach Diet–friendly?

Sugar alcohols, which are derived from plant products, are used in many sugar-free and low-carb products to provide texture and a sweet flavor. Common sugar alcohols include maltitol, mannitol, sorbitol, and xylitol. You'll see them in mints, gum, candy, syrup, and the like, often with the words "sugar-free" or "no sugar added" on the labels. Sugar-free products that contain sugar alcohols are not calorie-free (like sugar, sugar alcohols yield 4 calories per gram). The difference is that sugar alcohols evoke a low-glycemic response. They are digested more slowly by the body and, therefore, do not cause rapid fluctuations in blood sugar levels.

Products that contain sugar alcohols have been incorporated into the South Beach Diet under the "Sweet Treats" category, where you'll find items like no-sugar-added Fudgesicles and Popsicles. As you know, the South Beach Diet is not a calorie-counting diet, but we restrict "Sweet Treats" to 75 calories per day. The reason: Excessive amounts of sugar alcohols can cause GI distress such as bloating, gas, and diarrhea. The 75-calorie limit will help make sure you don't overdo it.

I'm on Phase 1 and have terrible headaches. What should I do?

Some dieters on Phase 1 experience headaches. To remedy this, make sure you eat three regular meals and *all* of your snacks. Snacks are mandatory during Phase 1—they help keep your blood sugar levels steady, and skipping snacks could cause headaches. Choose low-fat cheese, nuts, or another good source of protein when snacking.

Also check that your portions are not too small. This is a common mistake made by new dieters. Don't worry about counting calories. Instead, slow down, enjoy your meal, and give your stomach time to signal your brain that you're full. Additionally, if you recently limited your caffeine intake, you may be experiencing withdrawal headaches. If so, try adding back 1 cup of caffeinated coffee daily. Finally, be sure to drink plenty of water. Your headaches should subside over the next few days. If not, contact your doctor.

PHASE 2

Is the South Beach Diet safe for nursing mothers?

Check with your doctor before changing your eating habits while nursing. If your doctor gives you the go-ahead to start the diet, skip Phase 1 and start on Phase 2. Add an additional 3 cups of 1 percent or fat-free dairy to your daily intake.

You'll also want to make sure you're getting adequate amounts of vitamins A, D, B_6, and B_{12}—nutrients that are essential to your baby's development. Lactation experts suggest you take in an extra 500 calories a day during milk production. To determine your specific calorie needs, speak with your doctor.

Lastly, it's important to lose weight gradually—about a pound a week—because rapid weight loss could affect your milk supply.

I'm not losing as much weight on Phase 2. What should I do?

The rapid weight loss you experienced in Phase 1 will not and should not continue. Excessive weight loss in Phase 2 can result in the loss of lean muscle mass, which can ultimately lower metabolism. Plus, weight lost gradually is more likely to stay off.

Having said that, there are a couple of reasons why your weight loss stalled. First, you may be close to your optimum weight. At this point, any further weight loss would be cosmetic. Try increasing the length or intensity of your workouts to achieve your goals. Or maybe you're reintroducing high-glycemic carbs back into your diet too quickly. Be sure to add back carbs one at a time, paying close attention to how your body responds. Adding them slowly will keep cravings from returning and protect you from reversing weight loss.

What alcohol can I drink on Phase 2?

In general, people in Phase 2 can have one or two servings of alcohol a day. We recommend wine because it has antioxidants not contained in other alcoholic beverages. If you choose to drink, make sure you do so during or right after a meal, since a stomach full of food will slow the absorption of alcohol into your bloodstream—and keep your blood sugar levels steadier. And, of course, you'll want to avoid sugary mixers like fruit juices and regular tonic water—opt for diet tonic water instead.

Are there guidelines I should follow when buying bread?

When shopping for bread, it's important to read between the lines on the labels. Terms like "natural whole-grain goodness," "whole wheat" (as opposed to "100 percent whole wheat"), "multigrain," "enriched wheat flour," and "unbleached flour" may mean that the bread is actually made with refined flour, which is high on the glycemic index. Look for labels that say "100 percent whole wheat," "100 percent whole grain," or "100 percent whole grain rye." Choose breads with a high-fiber content—at least 3 grams per slice.

What do I do if my cravings return?

If your cravings return, it's possible that high-glycemic carbs have crept back into your diet. It could also be that you've added too many carbs back too quickly. Each person responds differently to

Phase 2's reintroduction of carbs, and you'll need to pay close attention to your reaction to different carb-containing foods. Choose a single food—like a piece of fruit or a slice of wholegrain bread—and add it to one daily meal for 1 week. Pay close attention to how your body responds over the next few days. Do you find yourself craving other carbohydrates or sweets? If the answer to either of these questions is yes, try a different type of carbohydrate and see if anything changes. When you find a carb that doesn't produce cravings, add a second choice and again monitor your reaction. Continue this process until you're able to eat 2 or 3 servings of good carbs a day. If you're really struggling, it may be helpful to return to Phase 1 until your cravings are back under control.

PHASE 3

What is the difference between Phase 2 and Phase 3?

During Phase 2, dieters continue to lose weight while learning to reintroduce carbs into their meal plans. It's a slow process that involves monitoring for the return of cravings. The goal is to reach your target weight while learning which carbs you can enjoy and which ones trigger cravings. Once you hit your target weight, you move to Phase 3—the maintenance phase. People in Phase 3 no longer need to follow any set meal plans; they simply apply the principles of the South Beach Diet and make good, healthy choices for life.

Now that I'm in Phase 3, can I eat anything I want?

Phase 3 is meant to be the maintenance phase of the South Beach Diet, and it's designed to last the rest of your life. Now that you've achieved your weight loss goals, it's time to incorporate the principles of the South Beach Diet into your daily eating habits. Phase 3 isn't about abandoning the diet and eating anything you want all the time—it's about making smart food choices. You focus on eating good carbs and good fats, but you'll find that you have a tremendous amount of freedom in choosing what you eat. Experiment with new recipes and ingredients, and know that your new lifestyle will greatly improve your overall health.

What should I do if I gain a little weight on Phase 3?

The South Beach Diet is designed to be flexible, and it also accommodates the occasional overindulgence. If you put on a few pounds, try returning to Phase 2 until you lose the weight. If your cravings start to return, you can also return to Phase 1 for a few days until you have them back under control.

What is the recommendation for omega-3s?

Omega-3s—polyunsaturated fatty acids that cannot be made by the body and, therefore, must come from the diet—have been shown to protect against stroke and heart disease. Most Americans don't get enough omega-3s in their diet. I recommend that you try to get between 3 and 4 grams of omega-3s daily.

To maintain a good intake of omega-3s, be sure to eat plenty of fatty fish (mackerel, tuna, and salmon, for example). Omega-3s can also be found in flax seed, canola oil, and fortified eggs. Fish oil supplements are another option. Be sure to check with your doctor before taking *any* supplement.

What are your recommendations for exercise?

I believe that regular exercise is an essential component of a healthy lifestyle. In addition to helping maintain weight loss, exercise offers a wide range of other health benefits. Find an exercise plan that you can easily incorporate into your existing lifestyle—you'll be more likely to stick with it. Aim for 30 minutes a day, and make it a mix of aerobic exercise (brisk walking, swimming), light weight training (which boosts metabolism and protects your bone density), and stretching. Check with your doctor before beginning any exercise routine.

HOW TO USE
THE FOOD GUIDE

The principles of the South Beach Diet are not difficult to comprehend, but in order to get the most out of the diet you also need to understand what comprises the foods you eat and how those foods fit in with the diet's principles. That's the purpose of this guide: to tell you what you need to know about more than 1,200 different foods and dishes.

Of course, we don't expect you to sit down and read this from cover to cover, as though it were a hot, new page-turner. So how can you get the most out of it?

One smart way to begin is just to browse the sections that hold some particular interest for you. If you love bread, for instance, we present four pages of information on various kinds. If you're a true blue carnivore, you can turn to the section on meat and find nine pages on how your favorites stack up.

You can also use this guide when planning meals. It's easy to flip from one category to another. We want to make it as effortless as possible for you to put together a healthy and delicious lifestyle, meal by meal. We've designed this book to be portable, so you can take it along when you're shopping for groceries or carry it to your favorite restaurant.

Foods are listed in alphabetical order, by category. For a serving of each, we give the following information:

Portion Size

On the South Beach Diet, you don't count calories, but that doesn't mean calories don't count. Be mindful of how much you're eating, especially when it comes to certain foods like nuts, where it's easy to eat two or three times the recommended portion size, and whole grain breads and other starchy foods that are reintroduced in Phase 2.

Total Carbohydrates

Although we provide this information, the South Beach Diet does not make you count carbs. I feel that learning about good carbohydrates is more important than tracking grams of carbs. By paying attention and eating the right carbs, you'll eat healthfully and lose weight.

As I've said before, the best carbohydrates are the unprocessed ones—those that provide fiber and are nutrient dense. These include whole fruits and vegetables and whole grain breads, pastas, and rice. Avoid refined carbohydrates that are packed with calories, sugar and/or fat, and usually offer very little nutrition: candy, pastries, white bread, instant rice, sugared cereals, and the like.

Total Sugar

Research shows that the average American presently eats about 33 teaspoons of sugar a day—per person! That's because many foods and beverages contain white sugar, corn syrup, and high-fructose corn syrup as one of their primary ingredients. All of these contribute to weight gain and should be avoided. Natural sugars, like those found in fresh fruits and low-fat dairy products, do not have the same effects on the body. That's why we recommended eating a variety of these foods in Phases 2 and 3.

Honey, molasses, and pure maple syrup are also natural sweeteners. They should be avoided in Phase 1, but may be used sparingly for flavoring in Phases 2 and 3. Brown sugar, while still a natural sugar, is processed by the body in the same way as white sugar and should be avoided.

Total Fat and Saturated Fat

We've also improved the information about the fat in foods. As you probably know by now, bad fats (such as saturated and trans fats) not only cause weight gain, but also can be hazardous to your overall health. These so-called "bad" fats clog your arteries and promote heart disease. But there are plenty of good fats, like the monounsaturated fats found in olive oil and canola oil, and the omega-3 fats found in fish, flaxseed, nuts, avocado, and green leafy vegetables. Starting with this edition of the guide, we give figures for both total fat and saturated fat for each food. The South Beach Diet doesn't ask you to count fat grams as part of your weight loss program; but for the sake of your heart health, keep your daily saturated fat intake below 10 percent of your daily calorie intake. This means that if you consume 2,000 calories a day, you should limit saturated fat to 20 grams or less.

We don't measure what are known as trans fats, which are used in many processed foods, for a very good reason: They're bad for you in any amount. In a packaged food, if you see "partially hydrogenated" before any of the first three ingredients, put that item back on the supermarket shelf.

Fiber

Fiber is a mainstay of the South Beach Diet. Dietary fiber, or what our grandmothers called "roughage," is the portion of edible plants that is not digested or absorbed from the small intestine. Most fiber comes from the structural parts of plants: the outer skin, stems, and leaves.

Plant foods commonly eaten by man include a wide variety of fruits, vegetables, grains, legumes (dried beans, peas, and lentils), nuts, and seeds. Removing dietary fiber is one of the worst things that one can do to a carbohydrate food, and it's the main way modern food processing turns a good carbohydrate (unrefined) into a bad carbohydrate (refined). We recommend that you look for at least 3 grams of fiber per serving when you eat foods like breads, rice, or pasta. To make sure you get the most fiber out of your whole fruits and vegetables, leave the skin on when possible.

Which Phase and How Often

The South Beach Diet is a three-step plan, going from the strictest early phase to the most liberal third one. As a result, some foods that are forbidden during the first 2 weeks are allowed later. Other dishes are out of bounds even during Phase 2, but are permitted in the third (maintenance) stage. We now tell you during which phase each food in this guide can be eaten, using four basic terms for each food: Good (G); Limited (L); Very Limited (V); and Avoid (A). Foods termed *Good* may be eaten regularly; *Limited* means it should be eaten no more than once a week; *Very Limited* means once every 2 or 3 months; and *Avoid* is pretty self-explanatory. We also use the term *Allowed (a)* for things like sparkling water or some sugar substitutes. Just to be clear, not all foods marked *Good* are created equal. Some foods, like non-starchy vegetables, can be consumed in larger portions than foods such as whole grain breads and low-fat dairy products. Use your South Beach Diet common sense.

But it's possible that the foods you are buying in your supermarket are different than what we've analyzed for this guide, even if it's the same *type* of food. So remember to read those labels! Watch out for canned foods thickened with

35

cornstarch or other starches, powdered mixes that contain trans fats, and sugar additives like high-fructose corn syrup.

These recommendations are guidelines, not hard and fast quantifiers, because so much depends on you as an individual. How often you might eat something is governed by which phase of the diet you are on, how much weight you're trying to lose, your body's own metabolism, and so on. The best way to use this guide is first to consult the allowable food lists for whatever phase you're on, and refer to any specific eating recommendations. Certain categories of foods like whole fruits are identified as "good" because they are, in fact, good, healthy foods; but if you're in Phase 1 of the diet, you still need to avoid them entirely. When you reintroduce more good carbs in Phase 2 and beyond, do so with discretion, paying attention to how your body responds. The South Beach Diet is not just a way of eating; it's a way of thinking about food. Once you understand its principles, you'll always be able to make the right food choices.

As we learn more, there will likely be changes in future editions of this book. To keep abreast of all changes and recommendations for the diet, visit www.southbeachdiet.com updates regularly.

BEANS AND LEGUMES

Beans and legumes are excellent sources of soluble fiber, which delays stomach emptying time, slows glucose absorption, and can lower blood cholesterol and assist weight loss. Beans are also an excellent source of protein for vegetarians. Soy protein, found in soybeans and soybean products, lowers LDL (bad) cholesterol. We recommend liberal consumption of these healthy foods.

Avoid canned beans that contain brown sugar, lard, or molasses.

BEANS/LENTILS

Food	Portion	Total Carbs (g)	Total Sugar (g)	Fat/ Sat Fat (g)	Fiber (g)	Ph 1	Ph 2	Ph 3
Aduki beans, boiled	½ cup	19	2	0/0	8	G	G	G
Baked beans								
Homemade, w/sugar	½ cup	27	11	6½/2½	7	A	A	A
Plain, vegetarian, canned	½ cup	24	4	0/0	6	G	G	G
W/bacon and brown sugar, canned	½ cup	29	13	3/1	7	A	A	A
W/beef, canned	½ cup	22	6	5/2	7	L	L	L
W/honey and mustard, canned	½ cup	31	12	0/0	7	A	A	A
W/pork, canned	½ cup	25	8	2/1	7	L	L	L
Black beans, canned	½ cup	17	1	0/0	6	G	G	G
Black-eyed peas, frozen	½ cup	20	3	1/0	4	G	G	G
Black turtle soup beans, presoaked, boiled	½ cup	23	4	0/0	5	G	G	G
Butter beans, canned	½ cup	18	1	0/0	5	G	G	G

BEANS/LENTILS (CONT.)

Food	Portion	Total Carbs (g)	Total Sugar (g)	Fat/ Sat Fat (g)	Fiber (g)	Ph 1	Ph 2	Ph 3
Calico beans, cooked	½ cup	24	2	0/0	9	G	G	G
Chickpeas, canned, drained	½ cup	27	1	1/0	5	G	G	G
Chickpeas (hummus) (homemade)	½ cup	25	2	11/1½	5	G	G	G
Chili, vegetarian, canned	½ cup	19	3	0/0	5	G	G	G
Chili, w/turkey and beans, canned	½ cup	13	3	1½/0	3	G	G	G
Chili con carne, w/beans, canned	½ cup	16	2	5/2½	5	G	G	G
Chili con carne, w/meat, canned	½ cup	11	1	12/4½	3	A	A	A
Kidney beans, red, canned, drained	½ cup	28	2	½/0	11	G	G	G
Kidney beans, white, boiled	½ cup	20	2	½/0	6	G	G	G
Lentils, brown, boiled	½ cup	20	2	0/0	8	G	G	G
Lentils, pink or red, boiled	½ cup	24	2	0/0	7	G	G	G
Lima beans, frozen, reheated	½ cup	18	2	0/0	5	G	G	G
Mung beans, cooked	½ cup	17	2	0/0	6	G	G	G
Navy beans, cooked	½ cup	24	2	½/0	6	G	G	G
Pinto beans, canned	½ cup	18	1	1/0	6	G	G	G

Food	Portion	Total Carbs (g)	Total Sugar (g)	Fat/ Sat Fat (g)	Fiber (g)	Ph 1	Ph 2	Ph 3
Refried beans								
Fat-free, canned	½ cup	24	1	0/0	7	G	G	G
Prepared w/corn oil	½ cup	20	1	5/1	8	L	L	L
Prepared w/lard	½ cup	24	1	6/2	7	A	A	A
Split peas, boiled	½ cup	21	3	0/0	8	G	G	G

SOYBEANS

Food	Portion	Total Carbs (g)	Total Sugar (g)	Fat/ Sat Fat (g)	Fiber (g)	Ph 1	Ph 2	Ph 3
Black soybeans, canned	½ cup	9	1	2/0	5	G	G	G
Green soybeans (edamame) boiled	½ cup	10	2	6/1	4	G	G	G
Yellow fermented soybeans (natto)	½ cup	13	3	10/1½	5	G	G	G
Yellow soybeans, boiled	½ cup	9	3	8/1	5	G	G	G

SPROUTS, BEAN

Food	Portion	Total Carbs (g)	Total Sugar (g)	Fat/ Sat Fat (g)	Fiber (g)	Ph 1	Ph 2	Ph 3
Kidney bean sprouts, raw	½ cup	4	1	0/0	1	G	G	G
Lentil sprouts, raw	½ cup	9	1	0/0	2	G	G	G
Mung bean sprouts, raw	½ cup	3	1	0/0	1	G	G	G

BEVERAGES

Most carbonated beverages are pure sugar and a source of empty calories. Diet sodas are okay in moderation, but water is the best choice for quenching thirst and hydrating your body. Both coffee and tea are major contributors of caffeine to our diets. Too much caffeine can cause a drop in blood sugar, leading to hunger and cravings. Try and limit your caffeine intake to 1-2 cups of caffeinated coffee or tea a day. Flavored coffees and mixes can be a source of hidden sugars.

Finally, research suggests that moderate consumption of alcohol reduces risk for heart disease and diabetes. We believe this is best accomplished by drinking red or white wine with meals. Beer is a less desirable choice because maltodextrins, the sugars in beer have higher glycemic indicies than table sugar. Cooking wines should be avoided because of their high sodium content. All alcohol is off limits in Phase 1.

BEVERAGES, ALCOHOLIC

Food	Portion	Total Carbs (g)	Total Sugar (g)	Fat/ Sat Fat (g)	Fiber (g)	Ph 1	Ph 2	Ph 3
Beers								
Lager	12 fl oz	6	0	0/0	½	A	A	V
Light	12 fl oz	5	4	0/0	0	A	V	L
Regular	12 fl oz	14	10	0/0	0	A	A	V
Liquors (gin, rum, vodka, whiskey)	1½ fl oz	0	0	0/0	0	A	L	L
Mixed drinks								
Rum and coke	1 standard recipe drink	26	26	0/0	0	A	A	A
Vodka and orange juice from frozen concentrate	1 standard recipe drink	30	29	0/0	0	A	A	A
Vodka and tomato juice	1 standard recipe drink	9	7	0/0	0	A	L	L

Food	Portion	Total Carbs (g)	Total Sugar (g)	Fat/ Sat Fat (g)	Fiber (g)	Ph 1	Ph 2	Ph 3
Wines, cooking								
Marsala	2 Tbsp	4	3	0/0	0	A	A	A
Red/white	2 Tbsp	1	1	0/0	0	A	A	A
Sherry	2 Tbsp	4	2	0/0	0	A	A	A
Wines, dessert								
Madeira	2 fl oz	8	5	0/0	0	A	A	A
Port	2 fl oz	8	5	0/0	0	A	A	A
Sherry	2 fl oz	1	5	0/0	0	A	A	A
Wines, table								
Burgundy	5 fl oz	2	2	0/0	0	A	a	a
Claret	5 fl oz	2	2	0/0	0	A	a	a
Red	5 fl oz	3	3	0/0	0	A	a	a
Rose	5 fl oz	2	2	0/0	0	A	a	a
White	5 fl oz	1	1	0/0	0	A	a	a
Wine spritzer	12 fl oz	3	3	0/0	0	A	a	a

BEVERAGES, NONALCOHOLIC

Food	Portion	Total Carbs (g)	Total Sugar (g)	Fat/ Sat Fat (g)	Fiber (g)	Ph 1	Ph 2	Ph 3
Carbonated drinks								
Club soda	12 fl oz	0	0	0/0	0	a	a	a
Cola	12 fl oz	40	39	0/0	0	A	A	A
Cream soda	12 fl oz	48	42	0/0	0	A	A	A
Ginger ale	12 fl oz	32	32	0/0	0	A	A	A
Ginseng-type soda	12 fl oz	39	39	0/0	0	A	A	A
Grape soda	12 fl oz	42	42	0/0	0	A	A	A
Lemon-lime soda	12 fl oz	38	38	0/0	0	A	A	A
Orange soda	12 fl oz	46	4	0/0	0	A	A	A

BEVERAGES, NONALCOHOLIC (CONT.)

Food	Portion	Total Carbs (g)	Total Sugar (g)	Fat/ Sat Fat (g)	Fiber (g)	Ph 1	Ph 2	Ph 3
Carbonated drinks (cont.)								
Pepper-type soda	12 fl oz	38	38	0/0	0	A	A	A
Root beer	12 fl oz	38	38	0/0	0	A	A	A
Seltzer water	12 fl oz	0	0	0/0	0	a	a	a
Soda, diet, artificially sweetened	12 fl oz	0	0	0/0	0	L	L	L
Sparkling mineral water	12 fl oz	0	0	0/0	0	a	a	a
Coffee, brewed								
Black, regular	8 fl oz	1	0	0/0	0	a	a	a
Black, decaf	8 fl oz	0	0	0/0	0	a	a	a
Coffee, cappuccino and espresso								
Cappuccino, prepared, w/milk	8 fl oz	7	7	4½/3	0	A	A	A
Espresso	1 fl oz	0	0	0/0	0	L	L	L
Coffee, instant								
Coffee substitute, cereal grain, prepared, black	8 fl oz	2	0	0/0	1	a	a	a
Flavored, international-type, sugar-free, prepared from mix	8 fl oz	3	0	1½/½	0	L	L	L
Flavored, international-type, w/sugar, prepared from mix	8 fl oz	8	8	3½/1	0	A	A	A

Food	Portion	Total Carbs (g)	Total Sugar (g)	Fat/ Sat Fat (g)	Fiber (g)	Ph 1	Ph 2	Ph 3
Dairy drinks and mixes								
Carob-flavored drink, prepared w/milk, from mix	8 fl oz	22	14	8/4½	1	A	A	A
Chocolate flavored drink, prepared w/2% milk, from mix	8 fl oz	30	30	3½/2½	1	A	A	A
Hot chocolate/ cocoa, prepared w/milk, from mix	8 fl oz	35	22	9/5	0	A	A	A
Milkshake, chocolate	12 fl oz	51	50	9/6	5	A	A	A
Milkshake, strawberry	12 fl oz	64	63	21/13	0	A	A	A
Milkshake, vanilla	12 fl oz	61	60	7½/5	0	A	A	A
Strawberry instant drink, prepared w/milk, from mix	8 fl oz	33	32	8/5	0	A	A	A
Strawberry instant drink, prepared w/water, from mix	8 fl oz	28	25	0/0	0	A	A	A
Juice-flavored drinks, sweetened								
Cranberry-apple or grape	8 fl oz	42	42	0/0	0	A	A	A
Cranberry juice cocktail	8 fl oz	36	36	0/0	0	A	A	A
Fruit punch, pouch-type	8 fl oz	30	29	0/0	0	A	A	A
Lemonade, homemade	8 fl oz	28	23	0/0	0	A	A	A

BEVERAGES, NONALCOHOLIC (CONT.)

Food	Portion	Total Carbs (g)	Total Sugar (g)	Fat/ Sat Fat (g)	Fiber (g)	Ph 1	Ph 2	Ph 3
Juice-flavored drinks, sweetened (cont.)								
Orange juice drink, prepared w/water, from instant drink mix	8 fl oz	31	23	0/0	0	A	A	A
Pouch-type, prepared	8 fl oz	30	30	0/0	0	A	A	A
Sports drink, Gatorade-type, w/glucose, ready to drink	8 fl oz	15	15	0/0	0	A	A	A
Soy milk shake, vanilla	12 fl oz	36	32	9/1½	0	A	A	A
Soy smoothie drink, banana	12 fl oz	36	30	4/½	0	A	A	A
Tomato juice, unsalted	1 cup	11	7	0/0	1	G	G	G
Vegetable Juice Cocktail	6 oz.	8	0	0/0	1	G	G	G
Teas								
Brewed tea, black	8 fl oz	1	0	0/0	0	a	a	a
Brewed tea, herbal	8 fl oz	0	0	0/0	0	a	a	a
Iced tea, instant, sweetened w/sugar, prepared w/water, from mix	8 fl oz	19	17	0/0	0	A	A	A
Iced tea, ready to drink, sweetened w/high fructose corn syrup, bottled	8 fl oz	22	17	0/0	0	A	A	A
Iced tea, unsweetened/diet iced tea	8 fl oz	1	0	0/0	0	a	a	a

BREAD AND BREAD PRODUCTS

Like grains, bread and bread products can be enjoyed often if you eat the right ones. Whole grain breads are the best choice. Whole grain products should read "100% whole wheat," "100% whole grain," or "100% whole grain rye." Watch out for breads that are labeled just "whole wheat" or "multi-grain." While some nutrients in these products may be preserved, their glycemic index is generally just as high as that of white bread. Look for at least 3 grams of fiber per serving. But remember, according to the guidelines for Phase 2, you do have to moderate your consumption of breads and starches once they are reintroduced to your diet.

Anything labeled "fortified" means that processing has removed essential vitamins and nutrients. Any attempts to return vitamins artificially are unlikely to be sufficient. Avoid "fortified" foods and commercial breads that include hydrogenated oils.

BREAD

Food	Portion	Total Carbs (g)	Total Sugar (g)	Fat/ Sat Fat (g)	Fiber (g)	Ph 1	Ph 2	Ph 3
Bagels								
Blueberry	3 oz (1 medium)	40	10	2/0	5	A	A	A
Cinnamon raisin	3 oz (1 medium)	49	2	1½/0	2	A	A	A
Egg	3 oz (1 medium)	47	1	2/0	2	A	A	A
Plain, onion, or sesame	3 oz (1 medium)	48	1	1½/0	2	A	A	A
Poppy seed	3 oz (1 medium)	48	1	1½/0	2	A	A	A
Whole wheat or multigrain	3 oz (1 medium)	48	2	1/0	8	A	V	L
Bread								
Baguette, white, plain	1 slice	12	0	1/0	0	A	A	A
Barley	1 slice	16	1	1/0	2	A	L	L

BREAD (CONT.)

Food	Portion	Total Carbs (g)	Total Sugar (g)	Fat/ Sat Fat (g)	Fiber (g)	Ph 1	Ph 2	Ph 3
Bread (cont.)								
Buckwheat	1 slice	14	1	1/0	3	A	L	L
Cinnamon raisin	1 slice	14	4	1/0	2	A	A	A
Cornbread, prepared from baking mix	3 in. square	41	4	9/2½	2	A	A	A
Cracked wheat, coarse	1 slice	14	1	1/0	3	A	G	G
Focaccia	1 slice	30	2	1½/0	1	A	A	A
French	1 slice	15	0	0/0	0	A	A	A
Gluten-free, wheat-free	1 slice	11	1	3½/0	1	A	V	V
High protein	1 slice	12	1	1/0	1	A	L	L
Honey oat	1 slice	15	2	1/0	2	A	A	V
Italian	1 slice	14	1	1/0	1	A	A	A
Multigrain, or 7-grain bread	1 slice	15	1	1/0	3	A	G	G
Oat bran	1 slice	11	1	1/0	3	A	L	L
Pita pocket, wheat, unleavened, 6"	1 each	35	1	1½/0	5	A	G	G
Pita pocket, white, unleavened, 6"	1 each	33	1	½/0	1	A	V	V
Potato	1 slice	14	1	1/0	1	A	A	A
Pumpernickel, whole grain	1 slice	13	1	1/0	3	A	G	G
Rice (white), low amylose	1 slice	11	0	2/0	0	A	L	L
Rice (brown), high amylose	1 slice	11	0	3½/0	0	A	L	L
Rye, light	1 slice	12	0	0/0	4	A	L	L
Rye, w/linseed	1 slice	15	2	1/0	5	A	G	G

Food	Portion	Total Carbs (g)	Total Sugar (g)	Fat/ Sat Fat (g)	Fiber (g)	Ph 1	Ph 2	Ph 3
Sourdough bread, rye	1 slice	15	0	1/0	3	A	L	L
Soy and flaxseed	1 slice	6	0	1/0	4	A	L	L
Sprouted wheat	1 slice	13	1	1/0	3	A	L	L
Stone-ground whole wheat bread	1 slice	13	3	1/0	3	A	G	G
Vienna	1 slice	14	0	1/0	1	A	A	A
White, enriched	1 slice	14	1	1/0	1	A	A	A
Whole wheat, made w/enriched wheat flour	1 slice	13	6	1/0	2	A	V	V
100% Whole wheat	1 slice.	13	2	1/0	3	A	G	G

BREAD PRODUCTS

Food	Portion	Total Carbs (g)	Total Sugar (g)	Fat/ Sat Fat (g)	Fiber (g)	Ph 1	Ph 2	Ph 3
Bread crumbs								
Dry, plain	¼ cup	19	1	2/0	1	A	A	A
Gluten-free, wheat-free	¼ cup	11	1	3½/0	0	A	V	L
Soft, white	½ cup	11	1	1/0	1	A	A	A
Breadsticks, plain	2 each	15	1	1/0	0	A	A	A
Bread stuffing, prepared	½ cup	22	3	9/2	3	A	A	A
Croutons, plain, dry	½ cup	21	1	2/0	1	A	A	A
Rolls								
Frankfurter/hot dog roll	1 each	20	3	2/1	0	A	A	V
Hamburger bun	1 each	21	5	2/0	0	A	A	V
Hoagie roll	1 each	62	5	9/5	3	A	A	A

BREAD PRODUCTS (CONT.)

Food	Portion	Total Carbs (g)	Total Sugar (g)	Fat/ Sat Fat (g)	Fiber (g)	Ph 1	Ph 2	Ph 3
Rolls (cont.)								
Kaiser	1 each	30	3	2½/0	1	A	A	A
Potato	1 each	28	4	2/½	1	A	A	A
Sourdough rye	1 each	29	1	1½/0	2	A	L	L
Whole grain	1 each	29	1	2½/0	4	A	G	G
Taco shell, baked	1 each	8	0	3/0	0	A	A	A
Tortilla, corn, unleavened, soft, 6"	1 each	12	0	½/0	1	A	A	V
Tortilla, wheat flour, unleavened, soft, 6"	1 each	22	0	3/0	2	A	L	L

BREAKFAST FOODS

Man was designed to consume much more fiber than we get in modern diets. Fiber slows our digestion and thereby helps prevent swings in our sugar and insulin levels. Both hot and cold breakfast cereals can be excellent sources of fiber; choose ones with a fiber content in the 6 gram or higher range. Hot oatmeal cereals are excellent but only those that are slow cooked; instant hot cereals have too high glycemic indices. And don't be fooled by cereals labeled "natural." Many types, including granola, have plenty of sugar and minimal fiber. Even worse, they may have hydrogenated oils.

Donuts are the worst breakfast choice. They have high levels of trans fats and highly processed flour with a very high glycemic index. Avoid store-bought muffins as well, because they are usually loaded with sugars.

CEREAL BARS

Food	Portion	Total Carbs (g)	Total Sugar (g)	Fat/ Sat Fat (g)	Fiber (g)	Ph 1	Ph 2	Ph 3
Atkins Morning (Creamy Cinnamon)	1 bar	14	0	8/5	6	A	G	G
Carbolite Crispy Caramel	1 bar	18	0	9/5	2	A	V	V

Food	Portion	Total Carbs (g)	Total Sugar (g)	Fat/ Sat Fat (g)	Fiber (g)	Ph 1	Ph 2	Ph 3
Milk and Cookies (Honey Nut Cheerios)	1 bar	26	16	4/1½	1	A	A	V
Nutri-Grain Blueberry	1 bar	27	13	3/½	1	A	A	A
Slimfast	1 bar	20	12	5/3	2	A	L	L
South Beach Chocolate	1 bar	15	7	5/3	3	A	G	G
South Beach Cinnamon Raisin	1 bar	15	7	5/2½	3	A	G	G
South Beach Cranberry Almond	1 bar	15	7	5/2	3	A	G	G
South Beach Maple Nut	1 bar	15	7	5/2½	3	A	G	G
South Beach Peanut Butter	1 bar	15	6	5/2	3	A	G	G
Special K	1 bar	18	9	1½/1	0	A	L	L

CEREALS, COLD, DRY

Food	Portion	Total Carbs (g)	Total Sugar (g)	Fat/ Sat Fat (g)	Fiber (g)	Ph 1	Ph 2	Ph 3
All-Bran	1 oz (½ cup)	22	5	1½/0	9	A	G	G
All-Bran, extra fiber	1 oz (½ cup)	23	0	1/0	15	A	G	G
Bran Buds	1 oz (⅓ cup)	23	8	½/0	12	A	L	L
Bran Flakes	1 oz (¾ cup)	23	5	½/0	5	A	L	L
Cheerios	1 oz (1 cup)	21	6	1½/0	3	A	L	L
Corn Chex	1 oz (1 cup)	26	3	0/0	0	A	A	A
Corn Flakes	1 oz (1 cup)	25	2	0/0	1	A	A	A
Corn Pops	1 oz (1 cup)	26	12	0/0	0	A	A	A
Crispix	1 oz (1 cup)	24	3	0/0	0	A	A	A

CEREALS, COLD, DRY (CONT.)

Food	Portion	Total Carbs (g)	Total Sugar (g)	Fat/ Sat Fat (g)	Fiber (g)	Ph 1	Ph 2	Ph 3
Fiber One	½ cup	23	1	1/0	14	A	G	G
Fruit Loops	1 oz (1 cup)	25	13	1/0	0	A	A	A
Frosted Flakes	1 oz (¾ cup)	26	12	0/0	0	A	A	A
Golden Grahams	1 oz (¾ cup)	24	10	1/0	1	A	A	A
Granola, homemade w/old-fashioned oats, honey, and almonds	1 oz (¼ cup)	17	6	5/2	2	A	A	V
Grape Nuts	1 oz (¼ cup)	23	3	½/0	2	A	A	A
Kashi, puffed	1 cup	23	1	1/0	2	A	A	A
Kashi, GoLean original	½ cup	20	5	½/0	7	A	G	G
Kashi, Medley	½ cup	19	5	1/0	2	A	L	L
Life	1 oz (¾ cup)	22	6	1/0	2	A	L	L
Muesli, Swiss	1 oz (¼ cup)	22	7	2/0	2	A	L	L
Puffed rice	1 oz (2 cups)	25	0	0/0	0	A	A	A
Puffed wheat	1 oz (2 cups)	23	0	0/0	3	A	A	A
Raisin Bran	1 oz (½ cup)	22	9	½/0	3	A	A	V
Rice Chex	1 oz (1¼ cup)	27	2	0/0	0	A	A	A
Rice Krispies	1 oz (1¼ cup)	24	2	0/0	0	A	A	A
Shredded Wheat	½ cup	20	0	0/0	3	A	G	G
Shredded Wheat & Bran	1 oz	23	0	0/0	4	A	G	G
South Beach Diet Toasted Wheats	2 oz (1¼ cup)	48	3	1/0	8	A	G	G
South Beach Diet Whole Grain Crunch	1 oz (¾ cup)	21	4	2½/0	4	A	G	G
Special K	1 oz (1 cup)	20	3	0/0	0	A	L	L

Food	Portion	Total Carbs (g)	Total Sugar (g)	Fat/ Sat Fat (g)	Fiber (g)	Ph 1	Ph 2	Ph 3
Total	1 oz (1⅓ cup)	21	4	½/0	3	A	A	V
Uncle Sam's cereal	2 oz (1 cup)	36	1	6/0	11	A	G	G

CEREALS, HOT, COOKED, PREPARED WITH WATER

Food	Portion	Total Carbs (g)	Total Sugar (g)	Fat/ Sat Fat (g)	Fiber (g)	Ph 1	Ph 2	Ph 3
Buckwheat groats	½ cup	17	1	½/0	2	A	G	G
Cream of Rice, instant	½ cup	14	0	0/0	0	A	A	A
Cream of Wheat	½ cup	13	0	0/0	0	A	A	A
Cream of Wheat, instant	½ cup	13	1	0/0	0	A	A	A
Farina	½ cup	12	1	0/0	0	A	A	A
Maypo	½ cup	16	4	1/0	3	A	A	A
Millet	½ cup	21	0	1/0	1	A	A	A
Oat bran	½ cup	13	0	1/0	3	A	G	G
Oatmeal								
Instant	½ cup	11	0	1/0	2	A	A	A
Old-fashioned	½ cup	13	0	1/0	2	A	G	G
Quick	½ cup	26	2	3/0	2	A	L	L
Steel-cut	½ cup	27	1	3/0	4	A	G	G

CEREALS, TOPPINGS

Food	Portion	Total Carbs (g)	Total Sugar (g)	Fat/ Sat Fat (g)	Fiber (g)	Ph 1	Ph 2	Ph 3
Almonds	6	1	0	4/0	1	G	G	G
Flaxseed, ground	1 Tbsp	3	0	3/0	2	G	G	G
Honey, pure	1 tsp	6	6	0/0	0	A	V	L
Oat bran, unprocessed	2 Tbsp	6	0	1/0	2	A	G	G

CEREALS, TOPPINGS (CONT.)

Food	Portion	Total Carbs (g)	Total Sugar (g)	Fat/ Sat Fat (g)	Fiber (g)	Ph 1	Ph 2	Ph 3
Psyllium seeds	1 Tbsp	6	0	0/0	4	G	G	G
Raisins	1 Tbsp	7	6	0/0	1	A	L	L
Rice bran, crude	2 Tbsp	7	1	3/½	4	A	L	L
Sugar	1 tsp	4	4	0/0	0	A	A	V
Wheat bran, unprocessed	2 Tbsp	5	0	0/0	3	A	G	G
Wheat germ	1 Tbsp	3	1	½/0	2	A	G	G

FAST FOOD BREAKFAST SANDWICHES

Food	Portion	Total Carbs (g)	Total Sugar (g)	Fat/ Sat Fat (g)	Fiber (g)	Ph 1	Ph 2	Ph 3
Biscuit w/bacon and egg	1 each	27	3	24/7	1	A	A	A
Biscuit w/bacon, egg, and cheese	1 each	31	3	31/10	1	A	A	A
Croissant								
W/bacon, egg, and cheese	1 each	24	3	28/15	0	A	A	A
W/ham, egg, and cheese	1 each	24	3	34/17	0	A	A	A
W/sausage, egg, and cheese	1 each	25	3	38/18	0	A	A	A
English muffin w/egg, cheese, and Canadian bacon	1 each	28	3	13/5	2	A	A	A

PANCAKES AND WAFFLES

Food	Portion	Total Carbs (g)	Total Sugar (g)	Fat/ Sat Fat (g)	Fiber (g)	Ph 1	Ph 2	Ph 3
Pancakes								
Buckwheat, plain, prepared from gluten-free batter mix, 6"	1 each	20	4	5/1½	2	A	A	V
Buttermilk, plain, prepared from batter mix, 5"	1 each	19	5	1½/0	1	A	A	A
Potato, homemade, 4"	1 each	22	1	12/2½	2	A	A	A
Whole wheat, prepared from batter mix, 5"	1 each	19	3	1/0	1	A	A	V
Waffles								
Belgian, frozen	1 each	29	7	7/1½	2	A	A	A
Blueberry, frozen, 4"	1 each	15	4	3/0	0	A	A	A
Buttermilk, frozen, 4"	1 each	14	1	3/0	0	A	A	A

PASTRIES

Food	Portion	Total Carbs (g)	Total Sugar (g)	Fat/ Sat Fat (g)	Fiber (g)	Ph 1	Ph 2	Ph 3
Apple bun, fat-free	1 each	43	22	0/0	0	A	A	A
Croissant, plain	1 each	26	6	12/7	1	A	A	A
Croissant, cheese, medium	1 each	27	6	12/6	1	A	A	A

PASTRIES (CONT.)

Food	Portion	Total Carbs (g)	Total Sugar (g)	Fat/ Sat Fat (g)	Fiber (g)	Ph 1	Ph 2	Ph 3
Doughnuts								
Chocolate	1 each	18	6	13/3	0	A	A	A
Chocolate, w/chocolate icing	1 each	34	17	22/6	1	A	A	A
Crème-filled, Bavarian	1 each	33	12	11/2½	0	A	A	A
Crème-filled, Boston	1 each	38	17	11/3	0	A	A	A
Cruller, glazed	1 each	51	30	16/4	1	A	A	A
Cruller, powdered sugar	1 each	38	12	16/4½	2	A	A	A
Éclair, chocolate, w/custard	1 each	21	12	13/3½	0	A	A	A
Glazed, mini, Munchkin-type	1 each	7	5	3/½	0	A	A	A
Jelly-filled	1 each	28	15	13/3½	0	A	A	A
Plain, w/chocolate icing	1 each	34	17	22/6	1	A	A	A
Plain, w/vanilla icing	1 each	33	19	24/7	0	A	A	A
Honey bun, glazed or iced	1 each	29	14	10/2½	0	A	A	A
Jelly-filled sweet roll	1 each	45	20	13/3½	2	A	A	A
Muffins								
Blueberry	1 small	27	11	4/1	1	A	A	A
Bran	2 oz	24	8	7/1½	2	A	V	V
Carrot	2 oz	26	8	1½/0	2	A	A	A
Chocolate chip	2 oz	26	8	7/2½	0	A	A	A
Fat-free	2 oz	26	14	0/0	0	A	A	A
Lemon poppy seed	2 oz	34	11	8/0	0	A	A	A

Food	Portion	Total Carbs (g)	Total Sugar (g)	Fat/ Sat Fat (g)	Fiber (g)	Ph 1	Ph 2	Ph 3
Muffins, English								
Cinnamon raisin	1 each	28	2	1½/0	2	A	A	A
Plain	1 each	26	2	1/0	2	A	A	V
Whole wheat*	1 each	27	2	1½/0	4	A	A	V
Scone, fat-free	1 small	14	4	0/0	5	A	A	A
Scone, regular	1 medium	26	6	9/2½	1	A	A	A
Sticky bun, cinnamon raisin	1 medium	43	20	14/2½	2	A	A	A
Toaster pastry								
Fruit-filled	1 each	37	17	5/1	1	A	A	A
Fruit-filled w/ frosting (blueberry)	1 each	37	18	5/1	1	A	A	A
Strudel, w/fruit	1 each	29	10	4/1	2	A	A	A

*Unless 100% whole wheat or whole grain

CANDY AND CANDY BARS

Most candy is pure sugar and as such should be avoided.

However, if you are going to indulge, a small quantity of dark chocolate is the best choice. The only negative about chocolate is its sugar content, and dark chocolate has a lower sugar content than other types.

There are now many varieties of low–carb, sugar-free, or diabetic candies on the market. Many use sugar alcohols such as sorbitol or mannitol as sweeteners. These sugar alcohols are sweet tasting, but instead of being absorbed into the bloodstream, they remain in the intestines. Consuming candy with high sugar alcohols can cause some stomach upset and diarrhea.

Food	Portion	Total Carbs (g)	Total Sugar (g)	Fat/ Sat Fat (g)	Fiber (g)	Ph 1	Ph 2	Ph 3
Almonds, carob-coated	1 oz	13	7	10/5	1	A	A	V
Almonds, milk chocolate-coated	1 oz	19	6	10/6	1	A	A	V

CANDY AND CANDY BARS (CONT.)

Food	Portion	Total Carbs (g)	Total Sugar (g)	Fat/ Sat Fat (g)	Fiber (g)	Ph 1	Ph 2	Ph 3
Candy corn	1 oz	26	26	0/0	0	A	A	A
Chocolate candy bar								
Plain	1½ oz	25	19	13/6	1	A	A	A
W/almonds	1½ oz	23	18	15/7	3	A	A	A
W/nougat filling	2 oz	46	28	6/5	1	A	A	A
Fruit candy, Skittles-type	1 oz	26	22	1/0	0	A	A	A
Fudge, chocolate walnut	1 oz	17	19	7/3½	0	A	A	A
Fudge, peanut butter	1 oz	22	15	2/0	0	A	A	A
Gum, sugar-free, w/sorbitol	1 stick	2	0	0/0	0	L	L	L
Gumdrops	1 oz	28	25	0/0	0	A	A	A
Gummy Bears	1 oz	28	25	0/0	0	A	A	A
Hard candy, Life Savers-type, peppermint	1 oz	28	18	0/0	0	A	A	A
Hard candy, sugar-free, artificially sweetened	1 oz	26	0	0/0	0	L	L	L
Jelly beans	1 oz	27	17	0/0	0	A	A	A
Marshmallows, regular-size	2 pieces	12	10	0/0	0	A	A	A
Milk chocolate candy kisses	1 oz	17	14	9/5	0	A	A	A
Dark Chocolate candy kiss	1 oz.	17	15	9/6	0	A	V	L
Peanut brittle	1 oz	22	19	3½/½	0	A	A	A

Food	Portion	Total Carbs (g)	Total Sugar (g)	Fat/ Sat Fat (g)	Fiber (g)	Ph 1	Ph 2	Ph 3
Peanuts, chocolate-covered, w/candy coating	1 oz	11	7	12/4½	2	A	A	V
Raisins, chocolate-covered	1 oz	19	17	5/3	1	A	A	V
Soy nuts, chocolate-covered	1 oz	14	12	8/4	4	A	A	V

CHEESE, CHEESE PRODUCTS, AND CHEESE SUBSTITUTES

Whole milk cheeses are a source of saturated fat, so choose low-fat or fat-free cheese for most of your eating and snacking. Two percent cottage cheese is the only 2% dairy product we recommend in Phase 1. Because of its high water content and the way it's made, one serving has less fat than 2% milk. Mozzarella cheese sticks make particularly convenient and healthy snacks. Occasionally, however, it's okay to enjoy a small amount of a very flavorful cheese such as blue cheese or Parmesan occasionally, because a little goes a long way to enhance the flavor of a dish without contributing a substantial amount of saturated fat.

CHEESE

Food	Portion	Total Carbs (g)	Total Sugar (g)	Fat/ Sat Fat (g)	Fiber (g)	Ph 1	Ph 2	Ph 3
Asiago	1 oz	1	1	8/5	0	L	L	L
Blue	1 oz	1	1	8/5	0	L	L	L
Brie	1 oz	0	0	8/5	0	A	A	V
Camembert	1 oz	0	0	7/4½	0	A	A	V
Cheddar								
Fat-free	1 oz	1	0	0/0	0	G	G	G
Low-fat	1 oz	1	0	2/1	0	G	G	G
Reduced-fat	1 oz	1	0	6/4	0	G	G	G
Regular	1 oz	0	0	9/6	0	A	V	V

CHEESE (CONT.)

Food	Portion	Total Carbs (g)	Total Sugar (g)	Fat/ Sat Fat (g)	Fiber (g)	Ph 1	Ph 2	Ph 3
Colby	1 oz	1	1	9/6	0	A	A	V
Cottage cheese								
Creamed, 4% milk fat	½ cup	4	3	5/3½	0	A	A	V
Fat-free	½ cup	6	5	0/0	0	G	G	G
Low-fat, 1% milk fat	½ cup	3	3	1/½	0	G	G	G
Reduced-fat, 2% milk fat	½ cup	4	3	2½/1½	0	G	G	G
Cream cheese								
Fat-free	2 Tbsp	2	0	0/0	0	G	G	G
Light, low-fat	2 Tbsp	2	2	2½/1½	0	G	G	G
Regular	2 Tbsp	1	0	10/6	0	A	A	V
Regular, whipped	3 Tbsp	2	2	11/7	0	A	A	V
Edam	1 oz	0	0	8/5	0	A	A	V
Feta	1 oz	1	1	6/4	0	L	L	L
Feta, reduced-fat	1 oz	1	0	3/2	0	G	G	G
Fontina	1 oz	0	0	9/5	0	A	A	V
Goat cheese, hard	1 oz	1	1	10/7	0	A	A	V
Goat cheese, soft	1 oz	0	0	6/4	0	L	L	L
Gorgonzola	1 oz	0	0	9/6	0	L	L	L
Gouda	1 oz	1	1	8/5	0	A	A	V
Gruyère	1 oz	0	0	9/5	0	A	A	V
Havarti	1 oz	1	1	8/5	0	A	A	V
Jarlsberg	1 oz	1	1	8/5	0	A	A	V
Limburger	1 oz	0	0	8/4½	0	A	A	V
Mascarpone	1 oz	1	1	13/7	0	A	A	V

Food	Portion	Total Carbs (g)	Total Sugar (g)	Fat/ Sat Fat (g)	Fiber (g)	Ph 1	Ph 2	Ph 3
Monterey Jack								
Fat-free	1 oz	1	1	0/0	0	G	G	G
Reduced-fat	1 oz	1	0	6/4	0	G	G	G
Regular	1 oz	0	0	9/5	0	A	A	V
Mozzarella								
Fat-free	1 oz	1	1	0/0	0	G	G	G
Part skim	1 oz	1	1	4½/3	0	G	G	G
Whole milk	1 oz	1	0	6/3½	0	A	A	V
Muenster	1 oz	0	0	9/5	0	A	A	V
Neufchâtel	1 oz (2 Tbsp)	1	1	7/4	0	L	L	L
Parmesan, hard	1 oz	1	0	7/4½	0	L	L	L
Parmesan/Romano, grated	1 Tbsp	0	0	2/1½	0	G	G	G
Provolone, reduced-fat	1 oz	1	0	5/3	0	G	G	G
Provolone, regular	1 oz	1	1	8/5	0	A	A	V
Ricotta, part skim	½ cup	6	0	10/6	0	G	G	G
Ricotta, whole milk	½ cup	4	0	16/10	0	A	A	V
Roquefort	1 oz	1	1	9/5	0	L	L	L
String cheese sticks (low moisture part-skim mozzarella)	1 oz	1	1	5/3	0	G	G	G
Swiss								
Fat-free	1 oz	1	1	0/0	0	G	G	G
Reduced-fat	1 oz	1	1	7/4½	0	G	G	G
Regular	1 oz	1	1	8/5	0	A	A	V
Yogurt cheese, low-fat	1 oz (2 Tbsp)	3	2	0/0	0	G	G	G

CHEESE PRODUCTS

Food	Portion	Total Carbs (g)	Total Sugar (g)	Fat/ Sat Fat (g)	Fiber (g)	Ph 1	Ph 2	Ph 3
American cheese, 2%, prewrapped	1 oz (1 slice)	1	1	3/2½	0	G	G	G
Cheddar cheese, extra sharp, cheese food	1 oz	3	3	7/4½	0	A	A	A
Cheez Whiz-type cheese sauce								
Light	2 Tbsp	6	4	3/1½	0	A	A	A
Regular	2 Tbsp	3	1	7/5	0	A	A	A
Squeezable	2 Tbsp	4	1	8/4	0	A	A	A
Jalapeño cheese, processed	1 oz	2	2	7/5	0	A	A	A
Pimiento cheese, processed	1 oz	2	1	9/6	0	A	A	A

CHEESE SUBSTITUTES (DAIRY-FREE)

Food	Portion	Total Carbs (g)	Total Sugar (g)	Fat/ Sat Fat (g)	Fiber (g)	Ph 1	Ph 2	Ph 3
Rice Cheddar cheese	1 oz	5	0	3/0	0	G	G	G
Soy cheddar cheese	1 oz	1	0	3/0	1	G	G	G
Soy cream cheese	1 oz (2 Tbsp)	1	0	8/2	0	L	L	L

CONDIMENTS

Some condiments can contain added sweeteners such as sugar, honey, corn syrup, and / or high-fructose corn syrup. Be sure to read the list of ingredients before you purchase.

Food	Portion	Total Carbs (g)	Total Sugar (g)	Fat/ Sat Fat (g)	Fiber (g)	Ph 1	Ph 2	Ph 3
Chili sauce, sweetened	1 Tbsp	4	4	0/0	—	A	A	V
Cocktail sauce, sweetened	1 Tbsp	3	2	0/0	0	A	A	V
Horseradish	1 tsp	1	0	0/0	0	G	G	G
Ketchup, sweetened	1 Tbsp	4	3	0/0	0	A	A	V
Lemon juice	1 Tbsp	1	0	0/0	0	G	G	G
Lime juice	1 Tbsp	1	0	0/0	0	G	G	G
Mustard	1 tsp	0	0	0/0	0	G	G	G
Salsa, homemade, w/oil	2 Tbsp	5	2	3/0	0	L	L	L
Salsa, ready-to-serve, no oil	2 Tbsp	2	2	0/0	0	G	G	G
Soy sauce	1 Tbsp	1	0	0/0	0	G	G	G
Steak sauce	1 Tbsp	5	3	0/0	0	L	L	L
Tabasco sauce	1 Tbsp	0	0	0/0	0	G	G	G
Taco sauce	1 Tbsp	1	1	0/0	0	G	G	G
Tartar sauce	1 Tbsp	2	1	4½/½	0	A	V	V
Teriyaki sauce	1 Tbsp	4	3	½/0	0	A	V	V
Vinegar	2 Tbsp	2	2	0/0	0	G	G	G
Worcestershire sauce	1 tsp	1	1	0/0	0	G	G	G

CRACKERS, DIPS, AND SNACKS

Most crackers and packaged snack foods contain trans fats and should be avoided. There are some 100% whole grain baked snack crackers that do not contain trans fats, and these can be eaten more liberally.

CRACKERS

Food	Portion	Total Carbs (g)	Total Sugar (g)	Fat/ Sat Fat (g)	Fiber (g)	Ph 1	Ph 2	Ph 3
Animal crackers	1 oz	21	4	4/1	0	A	A	A
Baked 100% Whole Wheat Crackers	1 oz.	19	0	5/1	3	A	G	G
Butter crackers, round-type	1 oz	18	3	7/1	0	A	A	A
Cheese crackers	1 oz	16	0	7/2½	0	A	A	A
Crispbread, rye	2 pieces	3	0	0/0	3	A	G	G
Graham crackers	1 oz	22	9	3/0	0	A	A	A
Matzoh	1 oz	24	1	0/0	0	A	A	V
Matzoh, whole wheat	1 oz.	22	1	0/0	3	A	L	L
Melba toast	1 oz	22	1	1/0	2	A	A	V
100% Stoned wheat crackers	1 oz	19	0	5/1	3	A	V	V
Oyster crackers	1 oz	20	0	3/0	0	A	A	A
Saltines	1 oz	20	0	3/0	0	A	A	A
Sandwich crackers, w/cheese filling	1 package	17	1	6/1½	0	A	A	A
Sandwich crackers, w/peanut butter filling	1 package	17	3	7/1½	0	A	A	A
Soda crackers	1 oz	20	0	3/0	0	A	A	A
Water crackers	1 oz	23	0	3/0	0	A	A	A

DIPS

Food	Portion	Total Carbs (g)	Total Sugar (g)	Fat/ Sat Fat (g)	Fiber (g)	Ph 1	Ph 2	Ph 3
Bacon and horseradish	2 Tbsp	3	1	5/3	0	A	A	A
Black bean	2 Tbsp	5	1	0/0	0	G	G	G
Blue cheese, reduced-fat	2 Tbsp	7	2	7/1	0	A	A	V
Chili and cheese	2 Tbsp	3	1	2½/1	0	A	A	V
Clam	2 Tbsp	3	1	4/3	0	A	A	A
Eggplant (baba ghannoush)	2 Tbsp	2	0	3/0	1	G	G	G
Guacamole, avocado	2 Tbsp	3	1	5/1	2	G	G	G
Hummus	2 Tbsp	4	1	2½/0	2	G	G	G
Nacho cheese	2 Tbsp	2	1	5/3	0	A	A	A
Ranch, reduced-fat	2 Tbsp	3	1	4½/3	0	A	A	V
Sour cream and onion	2 Tbsp	2	1	4/3	0	A	A	A

SNACKS

Food	Portion	Total Carbs (g)	Total Sugar (g)	Fat/ Sat Fat (g)	Fiber (g)	Ph 1	Ph 2	Ph 3
Bagel chips	1 oz	21	0	3/½	2	A	A	A
Banana chips, sweetened	1 oz	20	5	8/7	1	A	A	A
Beef jerky	1 oz	3	3	7/3	0	A	A	A
Caramel apple	1 medium apple	54	45	4/3	1	A	A	A
Cheese puffs or cheese curls	1 oz	15	1	10/2	0	A	A	A
Chex party mix, traditional	1 oz	18	3	5/1½	2	A	A	A

SNACKS (CONT.)

Food	Portion	Total Carbs (g)	Total Sugar (g)	Fat/ Sat Fat (g)	Fiber (g)	Ph 1	Ph 2	Ph 3
Corn chips	1 oz	16	0	9/1½	1	A	A	A
Cracker Jack, plain	1 oz	23	15	2/0	1	A	A	A
Fruit Roll-Ups-type, dried fruit snack	1 oz (2 pieces)	24	14	1/0	0	A	A	V
Popcorn								
Air-popped, plain	2 cups	12	0	0/0	2	A	G	G
Air-popped, w/1 tsp butter	2 cups	12	0	4½/2½	2	A	V	L
Air-popped, w/1 tsp oil	2 cups	12	0	5/0	2	A	V	L
Cheese popcorn	2 cups	11	0	7/1½	2	A	A	A
Microwave popcorn, plain	2 cups	17	0	7/2	2	A	V	L
Potato chips								
Fat-free	1 oz	24	1	0/0	2	A	A	A
Plain	1 oz	15	0	10/3	1	A	A	A
Potato sticks	1 oz	15	0	10/2½	1	A	A	A
Reduced-fat	1 oz	19	0	6/1	2	A	A	A
Pretzels								
Fat-free	1 oz	22	1	0/0	1	A	A	A
Hard, baked	1 oz	22	1	1/0	0	A	A	A
Low-fat	1 oz	22	0	1/0	1	A	A	A
Soft pretzel, w/mustard	3 oz	59	0	2½/½	1	A	A	A
Whole wheat	1 oz	23	0	½/0	2	A	A	A
Rice cakes								
Flavored	1 each	8	2	0/0	0	A	A	A
Plain	1 each	7	0	0/0	0	A	A	A

Food	Portion	Total Carbs (g)	Total Sugar (g)	Fat/ Sat Fat (g)	Fiber (g)	Ph 1	Ph 2	Ph 3
Tortilla chips	1 oz	18	0	7/1	2	A	A	A
Trail mix, traditional, w/raisins and nuts	1 oz	13	12	8/1½	1	A	A	A

DESSERTS

Desserts are fairly limited on the initial phase of the South Beach Diet, although you can feel free to enjoy sugar-free gelatin or one of our healthy and satisfying ricotta cheese combinations. Fruits, particularly berries, are ideal Phase 2 desserts. Strawberries dipped in dark chocolate are a personal favorite! Remember, the darker the chocolate, the lower the sugar content.

Many food manufacturers began adding partially hydrogenated fats—trans fats—to replace the previously used saturated fats in commercial goods as a way of preserving their shelf lives. Trans fats are common in cookies and baking mixes. Trans fats are worse than saturated fats and should be avoided as much as possible.

CAKES

Food	Portion	Total Carbs (g)	Total Sugar (g)	Fat/ Sat Fat (g)	Fiber (g)	Ph 1	Ph 2	Ph 3
Angel food cake	2 oz (⅙ cake)	33	17	0/0	0	A	A	A
Banana bread	2 oz (1 slice)	28	17	4½/½	0	A	A	A
Boston cream pie (sponge cake w/custard, no glaze)	3 oz (⅛ pie)	42	29	10/2½	0	A	A	A
Cake, plain, average, unfrosted	1 oz (1/12 cake)	34	18	4/1½	1	A	A	A
Cheesecake, chocolate	2¾ oz (1/16 cake)	30	23	20/9	1	A	A	V

CAKES (CONT.)

Food	Portion	Total Carbs (g)	Total Sugar (g)	Fat/ Sat Fat (g)	Fiber (g)	Ph 1	Ph 2	Ph 3
Cheesecake, plain	2¾ oz (¹⁄₁₆ cake)	18	17	18/11	0	A	A	V
Chocolate cake, from packet mix, w/ chocolate frosting	2¾ oz (¹⁄₁₂ cake)	43	38	13/3½	2	A	A	A
Chocolate cake, from packet mix, w/vanilla frosting	2¾ oz (¹⁄₁₂ cake)	40	30	13/3	1	A	A	A
Coffee cake, w/nuts	2 oz (3 inch square)	30	17	8/1½	0	A	A	A
Pound cake, made w/butter	2 oz (1 slice)	28	16	11/7	0	A	A	A
Sponge cake, plain	2 oz (⅛ cake)	35	21	1½/0	0	A	A	A
Vanilla layer cake, Pepperidge Farm-type	2¾ oz (⅛ cake)	35	25	1½/½	0	A	A	A
Yellow cake, from packet mix, w/ chocolate frosting	2¾ oz (¹⁄₁₂ cake)	43	24	14/3½	1	A	A	A
Yellow cake, from packet mix, w/vanilla frosting	2¾ oz (¹⁄₁₂ cake)	46	29	11/2	0	A	A	A
Flourless Chocolate Cake	2 oz (¹⁄₁₂ cake)	14	11	7/3½	1	A	A	V

COOKIES

Food	Portion	Total Carbs (g)	Total Sugar (g)	Fat/ Sat Fat (g)	Fiber (g)	Ph 1	Ph 2	Ph 3
Arrowroot biscuit	3 small biscuits (½ oz)	10	2	2/0	0	A	A	A
Butter cookie	2 cookies (1 oz)	19	6	5/3	0	A	A	A
Fig bar	1 bar (½ oz)	10	6	1/0	2	A	A	A

Food	Portion	Total Carbs (g)	Total Sugar (g)	Fat/ Sat Fat (g)	Fiber (g)	Ph 1	Ph 2	Ph 3
Gingersnap	3 small cookies (¾ oz)	16	4	2/½	0	A	A	A
Oatmeal	1 cookie (⅔ oz)	12	4	3½/1	0	A	A	A
Peanut butter, homemade	1 cookie (¾ oz)	12	7	5/1	0	A	A	A
Sandwich cookie								
Chocolate crème-filled	2 cookies (¾ oz)	15	9	4/1	0	A	A	A
Peanut butter crème-filled	2 cookies (1 oz)	18	10	6/1½	0	A	A	A
Vanilla crème-filled	2 cookies (¾ oz)	15	8	4/½	0	A	A	A
Shortbread	2 cookies (1 oz)	18	10	7/1½	0	A	A	A
Tea biscuit	2 biscuits (⅔ oz)	14	3	2½/½	0	A	A	A
Vanilla wafer	7 small wafers (1 oz)	20	10	5/1½	0	A	A	A

GELATIN

Food	Portion	Total Carbs (g)	Total Sugar (g)	Fat/ Sat Fat (g)	Fiber (g)	Ph 1	Ph 2	Ph 3
Sugar-free, prepared	½ cup	5	0	0/0	0	G	G	G
W/fruit, prepared	½ cup	18	17	0/0	0	A	A	A
W/sugar, prepared	½ cup	19	19	0/0	0	A	A	A

PIES

Food	Portion	Total Carbs (g)	Total Sugar (g)	Fat/ Sat Fat (g)	Fiber (g)	Ph 1	Ph 2	Ph 3
Apple fruit pie, two crusts	⅙ of 8" pie (4 oz)	40	21	13/4	2	A	A	A
Blueberry fruit pie, two crusts	⅙ of 8" pie (4 oz)	41	15	12/2	1	A	A	A
Cherry crumb pie	⅙ of 8" pie (4 oz)	47	28	13/3	0	A	A	A
Chocolate chiffon pie	⅛ of 8" pie (4 oz)	47	17	15/5	1	A	A	A
Chocolate peanut butter pie	⅛ of 8" pie (4 oz)	43	30	26/13	2	A	A	A
Peach fruit pie, two crusts	⅙ of 8" pie (4 oz)	38	18	12/2	1	A	A	A
Pumpkin pie	⅛ of 8" pie (4 oz)	31	16	1½	3	A	A	A

PUDDING AND MOUSSE

Food	Portion	Total Carbs (g)	Total Sugar (g)	Fat/ Sat Fat (g)	Fiber (g)	Ph 1	Ph 2	Ph 3
Pudding								
Bread pudding, homemade, w/cinnamon raisin bread	⅓ cup	21	15	5/2	0	A	A	A
Instant pudding, sugar-free w/reduced fat milk	½ cup	6	6	2/1	0	A	A	A
Egg custard, homemade, or no-bake recipe, prepared	½ cup	23	16	3½/2	0	A	A	A
Instant, prepared w/reduced-fat milk, chocolate	½ cup	28	21	3/1½	0	A	A	A

Food	Portion	Total Carbs (g)	Total Sugar (g)	Fat/ Sat Fat (g)	Fiber (g)	Ph 1	Ph 2	Ph 3
Instant, prepared w/reduced-fat milk, vanilla	½ cup	30	29	2/1	0	A	A	A
Rice pudding, homemade, prepared w/whole milk and long-grain rice	½ cup	30	19	4/2½	0	A	A	A
Tapioca pudding w/whole milk	½ cup	27	22	4/2½	0	A	A	A
Mousse								
Butterscotch, reduced-fat, prepared from mix	½ cup	10	1	3/3	0	A	A	A
Chocolate, reduced-fat, prepared from mix	½ cup	10	1	3/3	0	A	A	A
Mixed berry, reduced-fat, prepared from mix	½ cup	8	1	2½/2½	0	A	A	A
Vanilla, reduced-fat, prepared from mix	½ cup	8	1	3/3	0	A	A	A

EGGS, EGG DISHES, AND EGG SUBSTITUTES

The good news is that eggs are okay. It is true that eggs are high in cholesterol, but they are also low in saturated fat. Eggs are rich in protein and the yolk is a good source of natural vitamin E. Eggs do increase cholesterol minimally, but they also increase HDL, the good cholesterol. Omelets are a great way of including lots of healthful vegetables in your breakfast, while hard-boiled eggs have the advantage of being fast and convenient. If you don't like the yolk, egg white omelets made from Egg Beaters are good choices. So if you love eggs, go ahead and enjoy!

EGGS, FRESH

Food	Portion	Total Carbs (g)	Total Sugar (g)	Fat/ Sat Fat (g)	Fiber (g)	Ph 1	Ph 2	Ph 3
Extra large	1 each	0	0	6/2	0	G	G	G
Large	1 each	0	0	5/1½	0	G	G	G
Medium	1 each	0	0	4½/1½	0	G	G	G
Small	1 each	0	0	3½/1	0	G	G	G
White only (large egg)	1 large	0	0	0/0	0	G	G	G
Yolk only (large egg)	1 large	0	0	4½/1½	0	G	G	G

EGGS, OTHER

Food	Portion	Total Carbs (g)	Total Sugar (g)	Fat/ Sat Fat (g)	Fiber (g)	Ph 1	Ph 2	Ph 3
Duck	1 large	1	1	10/2½	0	A	A	A
Goose	1 large	2	1	19/5	0	A	A	A
Omega-3 fat enriched	1 large	0	0	4/1	0	G	G	G
Quail	3 each	0	0	3/0	0	G	G	G
Turkey	1 large	1	0	9/3	0	A	A	A

EGG DISHES

Food	Portion	Total Carbs (g)	Total Sugar (g)	Fat/ Sat Fat (g)	Fiber (g)	Ph 1	Ph 2	Ph 3
Boiled, 1 large	1 serving	0	0	5/1½	0	G	G	G
Deviled, 2 halves	1 serving	1	1	10/2½	0	G	G	G
Fried, 1 large egg w/1 tsp butter	1 serving	0	0	10/4	0	L	L	L
Fried, 1 large egg w/1 tsp trans-free margarine	1 serving	0	0	6/1½	0	G	G	G
Omelets, 2-egg								
Plain, w/1 tsp butter	1 serving	1	1	14/5	0	L	L	L
Plain, w/1 tsp trans-free margarine	1 serving	1	1	11/3	0	G	G	G
W/1 oz regular cheese	1 serving	1	1	19/9	0	L	L	L
W/1 oz regular cheese + 1 oz ham	1 serving	1	1	22/10	0	L	L	L
Extras: vegetables- 2 egg omlete	½ cup	4-5	2	10/3	2	G	G	G
Omelets, 3-egg								
Plain, w/2 tsp butter	1 serving	1	1	22/9	0	L	L	L
Plain, w/2 tsp trans-free margarine	1 serving	1	1	17/5	0	G	G	G
W/2 oz regular cheese	1 serving	2	1	34/17	0	L	L	L
W/2 oz regular cheese + 2 oz ham	1 serving	2	1	39/18	0	L	L	L

EGG DISHES (CONT.)

Food	Portion	Total Carbs (g)	Total Sugar (g)	Fat/ Sat Fat (g)	Fiber (g)	Ph 1	Ph 2	Ph 3
Omelets w/egg substitutes								
½ cup egg substitute w/1 tsp butter	1 serving	1	1	8/3	0	L	L	L
½ cup egg substitute w/1 tsp trans-free margarine	1 serving	1	1	5/1	0	G	G	G
Extras: ham	1 oz	1	1	8/2	0	G	G	G
Extras: reduced-fat cheese	1 oz	1	1	11/5	0	G	G	G
Extras: vegetables	½ cup	4-5	2	5/1	0	G	G	G
Pickled, 1 large egg	1 serving	0	0	5/1½	0	G	G	G
Poached, 1 large egg	1 serving	0	0	5/1½	0	G	G	G
Scrambled								
1 large egg, w/1 Tbsp fat-free milk + 1 tsp butter	1 serving	1	1	9/4	0	L	L	L
1 large egg, w/1 Tbsp fat-free milk + 1 tsptrans-free margarine	1 serving	1	1	6/1½	0	G	G	G
2 large eggs, w/2 Tbsp fat-free milk + 2 tsp butter	1 serving	2	2	18/8	0	L	L	L
2 large eggs, w/2 Tbsp fat-free milk + 2 tsp trans-free margarine	1 serving	2	2	12/3½	0	G	G	G

EGG SUBSTITUTES

Food	Portion	Total Carbs (g)	Total Sugar (g)	Fat/ Sat Fat (g)	Fiber (g)	Ph 1	Ph 2	Ph 3
Liquid	¼ cup	0	0	2/0	0	G	G	G
Powdered	⅓ oz	2	2	1/0	0	G	G	G

FAST FOOD

Most fast foods fall into the "avoid" category. They are dripping with saturated fats, trans fats, sugars, and empty calories. But there are ways to eat wisely, even at a fast-food restaurant: Choose broiled or grilled food over deep-fried foods, and choose burgers without all the toppings and special sauces. Look for the salad bar. When you go out for pizza, choose thin-crust vegetarian pizzas. The tomato sauce may play a role in preventing prostate cancer due to lycopene, an antioxidant found in tomato products.

FAST FOOD BURGERS, SANDWICHES, AND WRAPS

Food	Portion	Total Carbs (g)	Total Sugar (g)	Fat/ Sat Fat (g)	Fiber (g)	Ph 1	Ph 2	Ph 3
Bacon and cheese quesadilla	1 each	33	1	21/9	1	A	A	A
BLT soft taco	1 each	22	3	23/8	2	A	A	A
Burrito, bean (regular)	1	55	4	10/3½	8	A	L	L
Burrito, w/beef	1 each	39	2	19/6	2	A	A	A
Cheeseburger								
Double, w/condiments, on a bun	1 each	38	9	21/9	1	A	A	A
W/bacon, on a bun	1 each	35	10	36/14	1	A	A	A
W/condiments, on a bun	1 each	27	7	14/6	1	A	A	A

FAST FOOD BURGERS, SANDWICHES, AND WRAPS (CONT.)

Food	Portion	Total Carbs (g)	Total Sugar (g)	Fat/ Sat Fat (g)	Fiber (g)	Ph 1	Ph 2	Ph 3
Chicken Caesar Salad (without dressing)	1 each	17	2	9/3	3	G	G	G
Chicken Dipping Sauce								
Barbeque	1 pkt	11	9	0/0	0	A	A	A
Honey Mustard	1 pkt	3	3	4½/½	0	A	A	A
Ranch	1 pkt	1	1	13/2	0	G	G	G
Sweet-n-Sour	1 pkt	11	10	0/0	0	A	A	A
Chicken fajita wrap	1 each	51	3	20/5	3	A	A	A
Fish sandwich, breaded, on a bun, w/tartar sauce	1 each	41	5	23/5	1	A	A	A
Grilled chicken BBQ sandwich	1 each	34	7	3/1	2	A	A	A
Grilled chicken sandwich, w/mayonnaise (l T)	1 each	24	6	16/3½	2	A	A	V
Hamburger, w/condiments, on a bun	1 each	34	7	10/3½	2	A	A	V
Hot dog, on a bun								
Plain	1 each	18	4	15/5	1	A	A	A
W/chili and cheese	1 each	22	4	21/9	2	A	A	A
W/chili and sauce	1 each	24	7	32/12	2	A	A	A
Mandarin Chicken Salad (without dressing)	1 each	17	11	3/1	3	A	G	G
Nachos, w/cheese	1 each	34	2	18/8	1	A	A	A

74

Food	Portion	Total Carbs (g)	Total Sugar (g)	Fat/ Sat Fat (g)	Fiber (g)	Ph 1	Ph 2	Ph 3
Roast beef sandwich, on a bun, w/horseradish	1 each	35	7	14/7	2	A	A	V
Taco Salad w/o toppings	1 each	29	8	16/8	8	A	A	A
Tacos (regular-ground beef)	1 each	13	1	10/4	1	A	A	A
Subs 6"(whole grain bread)*								
Turkey	1 each	46	7	4½/1½	4	A	G	G
Roast Beef	1 each	45	8	5/2	4	A	G	G
Roasted Chicken Breast	1 each	47	9	5/1½	4	A	G	G
Ham (honey mustard)	1 each	53	9	5/1½	4	A	L	L
Turkey Breast & Ham	1 each	47	8	5/1½	4	A	G	G
Subs 6" (white bread)*								
Turkey	1 each	44	6	4½/1	4	A	A	V
Roast Beef	1 each	43	7	5/1½	4	A	A	V
Roasted Chicken Breast	1 each	45	8	5/1	4	A	A	V
Ham (honey mustard)	1 each	51	7	5/1	4	A	A	V
*includes lettuce, tomato, onion, green peppers, olives, and pickles								
Veggie Burger (no bun)		15	1	4/½	1	G	G	G

FAST FOOD BURGERS, SANDWICHES, AND WRAPS (CONT.)

Food	Portion	Total Carbs (g)	Total Sugar (g)	Fat/ Sat Fat (g)	Fiber (g)	Ph 1	Ph 2	Ph 3
Wraps (whole wheat tortilla)*								
Chicken, roasted	1 each	24	2	4½/1	2	A	G	G
Turkey	1 each	23	1	3/½	2	A	G	G
Ham	1 each	24	1	4/1½	2	A	G	G
Turkey Breast & Ham	1 each	24	1	3½/1	2	A	G	G
Wraps (white tortilla)*								
Chicken, roasted	1 each	20	3	5/1	0	A	A	V
Turkey	1 each	19	2	3½/½	0	A	A	V
Ham	1 each	20	2	4½/1½	0	A	A	V
Turkey Breast & Ham	1 each	19	2	4/1	0	A	A	V

*includes wrap, meat, green peppers, shredded lettuce, onions and olives

FAST FOOD CHICKEN

Food	Portion	Total Carbs (g)	Total Sugar (g)	Fat/ Sat Fat (g)	Fiber (g)	Ph 1	Ph 2	Ph 3
Breast, crispy	1 piece (5 oz)	16	0	25/6	0	A	A	A
Breast, extra crispy	1 piece (6 oz)	20	0	29/8	0	A	A	A
Chicken nuggets	4-piece serving	13	0	1½/½	1	A	A	A
Chicken nuggets	6-piece serving	20	0	17/4	2	A	A	A
Chicken nuggets	9-piece serving	29	0	25/6	2	A	A	A
Drumstick, crispy	1 piece (2 oz)	4	0	9/2	0	A	A	A
Drumstick, extra crispy	1 piece (2½ oz)	6	0	12/3	0	A	A	A
Popcorn chicken	3½-oz serving	21	0	23/6	0	A	A	A

Food	Portion	Total Carbs (g)	Total Sugar (g)	Fat/ Sat Fat (g)	Fiber (g)	Ph 1	Ph 2	Ph 3
Thigh, crispy	1 piece (3½ oz)	9	0	18/5	0	A	A	A
Thigh, extra crispy	1 piece (4 oz)	12	0	26/7	0	A	A	A
Wings, honey BBQ	6-pieces (5 oz)	14	7	11/2½	0	A	A	A
Wings, hot	6 pieces (5 oz)	3	0	14/3½	1	A	A	A

FAST FOOD POTATO ITEMS

Food	Portion	Total Carbs (g)	Total Sugar (g)	Fat/ Sat Fat (g)	Fiber (g)	Ph 1	Ph 2	Ph 3
Baked potato, large russet, w/skin, plain	10 oz potato	61	3	0/0	7	A	A	V
Baked potato, large russet, w/skin, w/sour cream	10 oz potato	61	3	3½/2	7	A	A	V
French fries								
Large order	1 each	73	1	33/7	6	A	A	A
Medium order	1 each	49	1	22/5	4	A	A	A
Small order	1 each	32	1	14/3	3	A	A	A
Mashed potatoes w/gravy	5 oz serving	23	3	6/3½	2	A	A	A

FATS AND OILS

With all the bad press fat has gotten over the last couple of decades, most Americans have concluded that just limiting fats makes a diet healthy. This was a major mistake. While limiting saturated fat (meat- and dairy-derived) and avoiding trans fats (manmade hydrogenated and partially hydrogenated oils) as completely as possible is important, the Mediterranean oils, including olive oil and omega-3 fish oils, appear to be good for both our blood vessels and our waistlines. We've given a "good" recommendation for Omega 3 oils and a "limited" recommendation for Omega 6 oils because the optimal ratio of Omega 6 to Omega 3 oils in our diet is 5 to1. Generally the ratio in the American diet is much higher. Omega 6 oils include corn, safflower, and soybean. There is no advantage to low-fat diet dressings that substitute sugars and starches for healthful oils. Along with a healthy oil, the vinegar in vinaigrette and oil-and-vinegar dressings is acidic and helps slow digestion. This lowers the glycemic index of the whole meal. Remember that nuts are also excellent sources of good fats and have been shown to help prevent heart attacks and strokes.

FATS

Food	Portion	Total Carbs (g)	Total Sugar (g)	Fat/Sat Fat (g)	Fiber (g)	Ph 1	Ph 2	Ph 3
Butter and margarine								
Light, 40% fat	1 tsp	0	0	1½/½	0	A	A	V
	1 Tbsp	0	0	5/1½	0	A	A	V
	2 Tbsp	0	0	11/3	0	A	A	A
Regular	1 tsp	0	0	4/2½	0	A	A	V
	1 pat	0	0	4/2½	0	A	A	V
	1 Tbsp	0	0	11/7	0	A	A	V
	2 Tbsp	0	0	23/14	0	A	A	A
	1 stick (½ cup)	0	0	91/58	0	A	A	A

Food	Portion	Total Carbs (g)	Total Sugar (g)	Fat/ Sat Fat (g)	Fiber (g)	Ph 1	Ph 2	Ph 3
Whipped butter, light	1 tsp	0	0	1/½	0	A	A	V
	1 Tbsp	0	0	4/2	0	A	A	V
	2 Tbsp	0	0	7/3½	0	A	A	A
Whipped butter, regular	1 tsp	0	0	2½/1½	0	A	A	V
	1 Tbsp	0	0	8/5	0	A	A	V
	½ cup	0	0	61/38	0	A	A	A
Butters, other								
Clarified butter (ghee)	1 Tbsp	0	0	13/8	0	A	A	V
	2 Tbsp	0	0	26/16	0	A	A	A
Garlic butter	1 Tbsp	0	0	11/7	0	A	A	V
Sweet cream butter, stick	1 Tbsp	0	0	11/7	0	A	A	V
Sweet cream butter, tub	1 Tbsp	0	0	9/6	0	A	A	V
Lard and animal fat								
Bacon grease	1 tsp	0	0	4½/1½	0	A	A	A
Light and reduced-fat spreads								
Benecol-type, light spread	1 Tbsp	0	0	5/½	0	G	G	G
Benecol-type, regular spread	1 Tbsp	0	0	9/1	0	G	G	G
Butter substitutes, butter buds or sprinkles	1 Tbsp	0	0	0/0	0	G	G	G
Cooking spray	2–3 second spray	0	0	1½/0	0	G	G	G

Food	Portion	Total Carbs (g)	Total Sugar (g)	Fat/ Sat Fat (g)	Fiber (g)	Ph 1	Ph 2	Ph 3
Country Crock-type, light	1 Tbsp	0	0	6/1	0	A	V	V
Country Crock-type, regular	1 Tbsp	0	0	11/1½	0	A	A	A
I Can't Believe It's Not Butter!-type, light	1 Tbsp	0	0	6/1	0	A	A	A
I Can't Believe It's Not Butter!-type, regular	1 Tbsp	0	0	10/1½	0	A	A	A
I Can't Believe It's Not Butter!-type, spray		0	0	0/0	0	G	G	G
Parkay-type, fat-free spray	1 Tbsp	0	0	0/0	0	G	G	G
Parkay-type, stick or tub, ⅓ less fat	1 Tbsp	0	0	7/2	0	A	A	A
Parkay-type, tub, light, soft	1 Tbsp	0	0	6/2	0	A	V	V
Trans-Fat Free Brummel & Brown-type, spread	1 Tbsp	0	0	5/½	0	G	G	G
Weight Watchers-type, light	1 Tbsp	2	0	4/1½	0	A	V	V
Mayonnaise								
Dairy-free (soy-based, eggless)	1 Tbsp	1	0	4/1	0	G	G	G
Fat-free	1 Tbsp	2	1	0/0	0	A	A	A
Light	1 Tbsp	1	1	5/1	0	L	L	L
Regular	1 Tbsp	0	0	11/1½	0	G	G	G

Food	Portion	Total Carbs (g)	Total Sugar (g)	Fat/ Sat Fat (g)	Fiber (g)	Ph 1	Ph 2	Ph 3
Miracle Whip-type salad dressing								
Fat-free	1 Tbsp	2	2	0/0	0	A	A	V
Light	1 Tbsp	2	2	3/0	0	A	A	V
Regular	1 Tbsp	2	1	7/1	0	A	A	V
Other fats								
Avocado	2 Tbsp	2	0	4½/½	2	G	G	G
Coconut, shredded, unsweetened	2 Tbsp	2	0	5/4	1	L	L	L
Light coconut milk, canned, unsweetened	1 Tbsp	0	0	1/½	0	L	L	L
Olives, green, stuffed	10 large	0	0	4½/½	0	G	G	G
Olives, ripe, black	8 large	2	1	4/0	1	G	G	G
Vegetable shortening								
Vegetable shortening, conventional-type	1 Tbsp	0	0	12/4½	0	A	A	A

OILS

Food	Portion	Total Carbs (g)	Total Sugar (g)	Fat/ Sat Fat (g)	Fiber (g)	Ph 1	Ph 2	Ph 3
Avocado	1 Tbsp	0	0	14/1½	0	G	G	G
Canola	1 Tbsp	0	0	14/1	0	G	G	G
Coconut	1 Tbsp	0	0	14/12	0	L	L	L
Corn	1 Tbsp	0	0	14/2	0	L	L	L
Cottonseed	1 Tbsp	0	0	14/3½	0	L	L	L
Grapeseed	1 Tbsp	0	0	14/1½	0	L	L	L

OILS (CONT.)

Food	Portion	Total Carbs (g)	Total Sugar (g)	Fat/ Sat Fat (g)	Fiber (g)	Ph 1	Ph 2	Ph 3
Olive	1 Tbsp	0	0	14/2	0	G	G	G
Olive, extra virgin	1 Tbsp	0	0	14/2	0	G	G	G
Palm	1 Tbsp	0	0	14/7	0	L	L	L
Palm kernel	1 Tbsp	0	0	14/11	0	L	L	L
Peanut	1 Tbsp	0	0	14/2½	0	L	L	L
Safflower	1 Tbsp	0	0	14/1	0	L	L	L
Sesame	1 Tbsp	0	0	14/2	0	L	L	L
Soybean	1 Tbsp	0	0	14/2	0	L	L	L
Sunflower	1 Tbsp	0	0	14/1	0	L	L	L
Walnut	1 Tbsp	0	0	14/1	0	G	G	G

FISH AND SHELLFISH

All fish is low in saturated fat, and many varieties of fish contain a good type of fat called omega-3. Omega-3, found in fish oil, appears to benefit us in several ways. As well as helping prevent heart attacks and strokes, there is evidence that fish oil helps prevent or treat depression, arthritis, colitis, asthma, and dry skin. It may also help us lose weight.

Shellfish, such as shrimp, were once labeled high in cholesterol, and avoided by people with concerns about their diets. But this has been proven wrong. Feel free to enjoy all shellfish on the South Beach Diet. However, the mercury content of fish is a growing concern. Canned tuna and swordfish should be limited for this reason and eaten no more than once a week.

FISH, BAKED OR BROILED

Food	Portion	Total Carbs (g)	Total Sugar (g)	Fat/ Sat Fat (g)	Fiber (g)	Ph 1	Ph 2	Ph 3
Bass, sea	3 oz	0	0	1½/0	0	G	G	G
Bass, striped	3 oz	0	0	2/0	0	G	G	G

Food	Portion	Total Carbs (g)	Total Sugar (g)	Fat/ Sat Fat (g)	Fiber (g)	Ph 1	Ph 2	Ph 3
Bluefish	3 oz	0	0	3½/1	0	G	G	G
Carp	3 oz	0	0	5/1	0	G	G	G
Catfish	3 oz	0	0	2/0	0	G	G	G
Cod	3 oz	0	0	½/0	0	G	G	G
Flounder	3 oz	0	0	1/0	0	G	G	G
Grouper	3 oz	0	0	1/0	0	G	G	G
Haddock	3 oz	0	0	½/0	0	G	G	G
Halibut	3 oz	0	0	2/0	0	G	G	G
Herring	3 oz	0	0	8/1½	0	G	G	G
Herring, kippered, smoked	3 oz	0	0	10/1½	0	G	G	G
Lingcod, greenling	3 oz	0	0	½/0	0	G	G	G
Mackerel	3 oz	0	0	12/3	0	G	G	G
Mahi mahi	3 oz	0	0	½/0	0	G	G	G
Monkfish	3 oz	0	0	1½/0	0	G	G	G
Ocean perch	3 oz	0	0	1½/0	0	G	G	G
Orange roughy	3 oz	0	0	½/0	0	G	G	G
Pike	3 oz	0	0	½/0	0	G	G	G
Pompano, Florida	3 oz	0	0	8/3	0	G	G	G
Salmon								
King, chinook	3 oz	0	0	9/2½	0	G	G	G
Pink, chum	3 oz	0	0	3/0	0	G	G	G
Red, sockeye	3 oz	0	0	7/1½	0	G	G	G
Smoked (lox)	3 oz	0	0	3½/1	0	G	G	G
Shark	3 oz	0	0	4/1	0	G	G	G
Smelt, rainbow	3 oz	0	0	2/0	0	G	G	G
Snapper	3 oz	0	0	1/0	0	G	G	G

FISH, BAKED OR BROILED (CONT.)

Food	Portion	Total Carbs (g)	Total Sugar (g)	Fat/ Sat Fat (g)	Fiber (g)	Ph 1	Ph 2	Ph 3
Sole	3 oz	0	0	1/0	0	G	G	G
Sturgeon	3 oz	0	0	3½/1	0	G	G	G
Swordfish	3 oz	0	0	3½/1	0	G	G	G
Trout, rainbow	3 oz	0	0	4½/1½	0	G	G	G
Trout, sea	3 oz	0	0	3/1	0	G	G	G
Tuna, fresh	3 oz	0	0	4/1	0	G	G	G
Turbot	3 oz	0	0	3/0	0	G	G	G
Whitefish, smoked	3 oz	0	0	1/0	0	G	G	G
Whiting	3 oz	0	0	1/0	0	G	G	G
Yellowtail	3 oz	0	0	4½/1	0	G	G	G

FISH, BREADED

Food	Portion	Total Carbs (g)	Total Sugar (g)	Fat/ Sat Fat (g)	Fiber (g)	Ph 1	Ph 2	Ph 3
Clams, fried	3 oz	10	2	9/2½	0	A	A	A
Fish fillet, frozen, oven baked	3 oz	14	2	15/2	0	A	A	A
Fish sticks, frozen, oven baked	3 oz	20	2	10/2½	1	A	A	A
Oysters, fried	3 oz	10	0	11/2½	0	A	A	A
Scallops, fried	3 oz	11	1	10/2	0	A	A	A
Shrimp, fried	3 oz	10	0	10/2	0	A	A	A

FISH, CANNED

Food	Portion	Total Carbs (g)	Total Sugar (g)	Fat/ Sat Fat (g)	Fiber (g)	Ph 1	Ph 2	Ph 3
Anchovies, in oil, drained	3 oz	0	0	8/2	0	G	G	G
Salmon, pink, drained	3 oz	0	0	5/1½	0	G	G	G
Sardines								
In mustard sauce, drained	3 oz	0	0	10/2½	0	G	G	G
In oil, drained	3 oz	0	0	10/1½	0	G	G	G
In tomato sauce, drained	3 oz	0	0	9/2½	0	G	G	G
In water. skinless	3 oz	0	0	1½½	0	G	G	G
Tuna								
Light, in oil, drained	3 oz	0	0	7/1½	0	G	G	G
Light, in water, drained	3 oz	0	0	½/0	0	G	G	G
White, in oil, drained	3 oz	0	0	7/1	0	G	G	G
White, in water, drained	3 oz	0	0	2½/½	0	G	G	G

SHELLFISH, COOKED

Food	Portion	Total Carbs (g)	Total Sugar (g)	Fat/ Sat Fat (g)	Fiber (g)	Ph 1	Ph 2	Ph 3
Clams	1 dozen (3 oz)	0	0	1/0	0	G	G	G
Crab								
Blue, soft-shell	3 oz	0	0	1/0	0	G	G	G
Dungeness	3 oz	0	0	1/0	0	G	G	G
King, leg	3 oz	0	0	½/0	0	G	G	G

SHELLFISH, COOKED (CONT.)

Food	Portion	Total Carbs (g)	Total Sugar (g)	Fat/ Sat Fat (g)	Fiber (g)	Ph 1	Ph 2	Ph 3
Crayfish	3 oz	0	0	1/0	0	G	G	G
Lobster	3 oz	0	0	1/0	0	G	G	G
Mussels	3 oz	0	0	2/0	0	G	G	G
Oysters	6 medium (3 oz)	0	0	1½/0	0	G	G	G
Scallops	3 oz	0	0	½/0	0	G	G	G
Shrimp	3 oz	0	0	1½/0	0	G	G	G

FRUIT AND FRUIT JUICES

Because of their carbohydrate, fiber, vitamin, and mineral content, most fruits can be eaten frequently after Phase 1. There are some that are high in sugar and should be eaten in limited amounts. We encourage the consumption of whole fruit. Avoid canned fruits packed in heavy syrup and processed commercial fruit juices. Commercial fruit juices are frequently concentrates of the fruit's sugar without any of the fiber. You get much more nutritional benefit out of eating a whole fruit. If you need your glass of OJ in the morning, fresh squeezed is best.

FRUIT, CANNED

Food	Portion	Total Carbs (g)	Total Sugar (g)	Fat/ Sat Fat (g)	Fiber (g)	Ph 1	Ph 2	Ph 3
Apricots, in light syrup	½ cup	21	17	0/0	2	A	V	V
Fruit cocktail, in natural juices	½ cup	15	13	0/0	1	A	V	V
Peaches								
In heavy syrup	½ cup	26	23	0/0	2	A	A	A
In light syrup	½ cup	18	17	0/0	2	A	V	V
In natural juices	½ cup	14	13	0/0	2	A	V	L

Food	Portion	Total Carbs (g)	Total Sugar (g)	Fat/ Sat Fat (g)	Fiber (g)	Ph 1	Ph 2	Ph 3
Pear halves, in light syrup	½ cup	19	15	0/0	2	A	V	V
Pear halves, in natural juices	½ cup	16	12	0/0	2	A	V	V

FRUIT, DRIED

Food	Portion	Total Carbs (g)	Total Sugar (g)	Fat/ Sat Fat (g)	Fiber (g)	Ph 1	Ph 2	Ph 3
Apples	1 oz	19	16	0/0	2	A	G	G
Apricots	1 oz	18	12	0/0	1	A	G	G
Currants	1 oz	21	19	0/0	2	A	A	V
Dates, pitted	1 oz	21	18	0/0	2	A	A	V
Figs	1 oz	18	14	0/0	3	A	V	L
Prunes, pitted	1 oz	18	12	0/0	2	A	L	G
Raisins	1 oz	22	18	0/0	2	A	V	L

FRUIT, FRESH

Food	Portion	Total Carbs (g)	Total Sugar (g)	Fat/ Sat Fat (g)	Fiber (g)	Ph 1	Ph 2	Ph 3
Apple	1 small (4 oz)	17	15	0/0	2	A	G	G
Applesauce, unsweetened	½ cup	14	12	0/0	2	A	L	L
Apricots	3 small (5 oz)	16	13	0/0	3	A	G	G
Banana, ripe	1 small (3½ oz)	23	12	0/0	3	A	G	G
Blueberries	¾ cup	16	11	0/0	3	A	G	G
Cantaloupe, melon	1 cup	13	12	0/0	1	A	G	G
Cherries, sour, pitted	1 cup	19	13	0/0	2	A	G	G

FRUIT, FRESH (CONT.)

Food	Portion	Total Carbs (g)	Total Sugar (g)	Fat/ Sat Fat (g)	Fiber (g)	Ph 1	Ph 2	Ph 3
Cherries, sweet, pitted	1 cup	24	21	0/0	3	A	L	L
Cranberries	½ cup	6	2	0/0	2	A	G	G
Grapefruit	½ large	13	12	0/0	2	A	G	G
Grapes, red or green	1 cup (3¼ oz, 20 grapes)	16	15	0/0	0	A	G	G
Kiwi	1 med. (3 oz)	12	8	0/0	3	A	G	G
Lemon	1 med. (3 oz)	5	1	0/0	2	G	G	G
Lime	1 med. (3 oz)	7	0	0/0	2	G	G	G
Mango	1 small (3½ oz)	17	15	½/0	2	A	G	G
Nectarine	1 small (5 oz)	16	12	½/0	2	A	G	G
Orange	1 small (6 oz)	20	16	0/0	4	A	G	G
Papaya	1 small (8 oz)	22	13	0/0	4	A	G	G
Peach	1 med. (4 oz)	11	9	0/0	2	A	G	G
Pear	1 med. (4 oz)	18	11	0/0	4	A	G	G
Pineapple	1 cup	20	14	0/0	2	A	L	L
Plum	2 small (5 oz)	20	11	1/0	2	A	G	G
Raspberries	1 cup	15	5	1/0	8	A	G	G
Strawberries (whole)	1 cup	11	7	0/0	3	A	G	G
Tangerine	1 med. (4 oz)	15	12	0/0	2	A	G	G
Watermelon	1 cup	12	10	0/0	0	A	V	V

FRUIT JUICES, UNSWEETENED

Food	Portion	Total Carbs (g)	Total Sugar (g)	Fat/ Sat Fat (g)	Fiber (g)	Ph 1	Ph 2	Ph 3
Apple cider	½ cup	15	13	0/0	0	A	A	L
Apple juice	½ cup	14	14	0/0	0	A	A	L
Apricot nectar	½ cup	18	17	0/0	0	A	A	V
Grape juice	½ cup	16	16	0/0	0	A	A	L
Grapefruit juice, fresh	½ cup	12	11	0/0	0	A	V	L
Mango nectar	½ cup	19	18	0/0	0	A	A	V
Orange juice, fresh	½ cup	13	10	0/0	0	A	V	L
Orange juice, reconstituted from frozen concentrate	½ cup	13	10	0/0	0	A	A	V
Papaya nectar	½ cup	18	17	0/0	0	A	A	V
Peach nectar	½ cup	17	17	0/0	0	A	A	V
Pear nectar	½ cup	20	19	0/0	0	A	A	V
Pineapple juice	½ cup	15	12	0/0	0	A	A	V
Prune juice	½ cup	21	8	0/0	2	A	V	L

GRAINS AND RICE

Enjoy grains frequently, as long as you eat the right ones. The more intact the grain, the higher the fiber and nutrition. Whole grains, including wheat, rye, barley, corn, and some types of rice, are rich in bran, B vitamins, iron, and other minerals. Stay away from white rice, which is milled, removing the bran and germ. Brown rice is a much better source of B vitamins, minerals, and fiber. Wild rice is frequently served in combination with white or brown rice and is very nutritious and low on the glycemic index. Couscous is another good choice to substitute for white rice or white potatoes.

GRAINS, COOKED

Food	Portion	Total Carbs (g)	Total Sugar (g)	Fat/ Sat Fat (g)	Fiber (g)	Ph 1	Ph 2	Ph 3
Amaranth	½ cup	32	1	3/1	7	A	G	G
Barley, pearled	½ cup	22	0	0/0	3	A	G	G
Buckwheat (kasha)	½ cup	17	1	½/0	2	A	G	G
Bulgur	½ cup	17	0	0/0	4	A	G	G
Corn grits	½ cup	16	0	0/0	0	A	A	V
Cornmeal	½ cup	12	0	½/0	1	A	A	V
Couscous	½ cup	18	0	0/0	1	A	G	G
Millet	½ cup	21	0	1/0	1	A	A	A
Oats, whole kernel	½ cup	26	1	3/0	4	A	G	G
Rye, whole kernel	½ cup	34	2	1/0	6	A	G	G
Wheat, whole kernel	½ cup	32	0	½/0	5	A	G	G

RICE, COOKED

Food	Portion	Total Carbs (g)	Total Sugar (g)	Fat/ Sat Fat (g)	Fiber (g)	Ph 1	Ph 2	Ph 3
Arborio risotto	½ cup	24	0	0/0	0	A	A	A
Basmati	½ cup	23	0	0/0	0	A	V	L

Food	Portion	Total Carbs (g)	Total Sugar (g)	Fat/ Sat Fat (g)	Fiber (g)	Ph 1	Ph 2	Ph 3
Brown	½ cup	22	0	1/0	2	A	G	G
Brown, par-boiled (converted)	½ cup	23	0	½/0	2	A	G	G
Glutinous	½ cup	18	0	0/0	0	A	A	A
Jasmine	½ cup	18	0	0/0	0	A	A	A
White, instant	½ cup	18	0	0/0	0	A	A	A
White, long-grain	½ cup	22	0	0/0	0	A	V	V
White, long-grain, converted-type	½ cup	22	0	0/0	0	A	V	V
Wild	½ cup	35	1	0/0	2	A	G	G

GRAVIES AND SAUCES

Canned or prepackaged gravies and sauces are often very high in sodium and fat, so read the labels carefully. When serving meat, stick to the natural, de-fatted meat juices.

GRAVIES

Food	Portion	Total Carbs (g)	Total Sugar (g)	Fat/ Sat Fat (g)	Fiber (g)	Ph 1	Ph 2	Ph 3
Au jus	¼ cup	1	0	0/0	0	G	G	G
Beef, mushroom, or turkey, canned	¼ cup	3	0	1½/½	0	A	V	V
Beef, turkey, or chicken, fat-free, canned	¼ cup	5	0	0/0	0	A	V	V
Chicken, canned	¼ cup	3	0	3½/1	0	A	V	V
Homemade, thick	¼ cup	22	2	21/5	0	A	A	A
Mix, brown, prepared w/water	¼ cup	3	0	0/0	0	A	V	V

SAUCES

Food	Portion	Total Carbs (g)	Total Sugar (g)	Fat/ Sat Fat (g)	Fiber (g)	Ph 1	Ph 2	Ph 3
Alfredo	¼ cup	3	2	18/7	0	A	A	A
Béarnaise	¼ cup	1	1	17/10	0	A	A	A
Béchamel (white sauce), thin, homemade	¼ cup	3	2	6/3½	0	A	A	V
Bordelaise	¼ cup	5	1	6/3½	0	A	V	V
Cheese fondue, homemade	¼ cup	2	0	7/4½	0	A	A	V
Clam, red	¼ cup	4	2	½/0	0	G	G	G
Clam, white	¼ cup	2	1	5/½	0	G	G	G
Hollandaise	¼ cup	1	1	18/10	0	A	A	A
Marinara	¼ cup	7	6	1½/0	0	G	G	G
Mornay	¼ cup	6	3	15/7	0	A	A	A
Peanut	¼ cup	6	2	1½	1	G	G	G
Pizza, unsweetened	¼ cup	5	3	0/0	1	G	G	G

ICE CREAM AND FROZEN DESSERTS

Ice cream is not a part of the South Beach Diet, although you can enjoy a small amount as a *very* occasional treat. Opt for sugar-free fudge or fruit pops instead.

ICE CREAM

Food	Portion	Total Carbs (g)	Total Sugar (g)	Fat/ Sat Fat (g)	Fiber (g)	Ph 1	Ph 2	Ph 3
Low-fat								
Neapolitan, no sugar added	½ cup	15	4	4/2½	3	A	A	V
Vanilla, 50% less fat	½ cup	17	15	3/2	0	A	A	V

Food	Portion	Total Carbs (g)	Total Sugar (g)	Fat/ Sat Fat (g)	Fiber (g)	Ph 1	Ph 2	Ph 3
Premium								
Butter pecan	½ cup	14	13	12/5	0	A	A	V
Cookies and cream	½ cup	20	17	10/6	0	A	A	V
French vanilla, light	½ cup	18	14	4/2	0	A	A	V
Macadamia nut	½ cup	20	18	24/12	0	A	A	V
Mint chocolate chip	½ cup	25	22	20/11	1	A	A	V
Regular								
Chocolate	½ cup	17	16	8/5	1	A	A	V
Peach	½ cup	17	16	6/4	0	A	A	V
Strawberry	½ cup	15	15	7/4	0	A	A	V
Vanilla	½ cup	14	14	10/6	0	A	A	V

ICE CREAM BARS AND POPS

Food	Portion	Total Carbs (g)	Total Sugar (g)	Fat/ Sat Fat (g)	Fiber (g)	Ph 1	Ph 2	Ph 3
Fudge pop, no sugar added	1 each	9	2	0/0	0	G	G	G
Ice cream sandwich	1 each	22	15	6/3	0	A	A	V
Juice bar, fruit-juice sweetened (Dole)	1 each	16	16	0/0	1	A	A	V
Klondike-type bar (3½ oz.)	1 each	24	19	19/19	0	A	A	V
Nutty Buddy-type cone	1 each	22	16	14/6	1	A	A	A
Popsicle-type, sugar-free	1 each	3	0	0/0	0	G	G	G

FROZEN DESSERTS

Food	Portion	Total Carbs (g)	Total Sugar (g)	Fat/ Sat Fat (g)	Fiber (g)	Ph 1	Ph 2	Ph 3
Frozen yogurt								
Chocolate, fat-free	½ cup	21	16	0/0	1	A	A	V
Chocolate, low-fat	½ cup	21	17	2/1	1	A	A	V
Chocolate, regular	½ cup	21	17	5/3	2	A	A	V
Vanilla or fruit, low-fat	½ cup	17	17	1½/1	0	A	A	V
Vanilla or fruit, regular	½ cup	21	16	4½/3	0	A	A	V
Ice milk, vanilla, chocolate, or strawberry	½ cup	17	16	2/1½	0	A	A	V
Snow cone, w/syrup, flavored	6 oz cone	64	16	0/0	0	A	A	A
Tofu-based frozen dessert	½ cup	22	15	10/4	0	A	A	V

MEAL REPLACEMENT BARS AND SHAKES

Meal replacement bars and shakes were created to fill the need for a quick meal for people on the run who are trying to lose weight. Usually the bars contain 170–300 calories, so they're more than a snack. They do contain protein, fiber, and other nutrients, and many are low in fat and saturated fat. However, some have as much fat and saturated fat as a chocolate bar, and some are extremely high in sugar as well.

The South Beach Diet encourages eating healthy meals based on whole foods. But, when circumstances do not permit, a meal replacement bar or beverage can be quite useful; certainly, a good meal replacement bar is preferable to fast food.

BARS

Food	Portion	Total Carbs (g)	Total Sugar (g)	Fat/ Sat Fat (g)	Fiber (g)	Ph 1	Ph 2	Ph 3
Atkins Advantage, chocolate peanut butter	1 bar	21	1	12/6	10	A	L	L
Balance Gold (average)	1 bar	22	11	7/4	1	A	A	V
Carb Solution, chocolate peanut butter	1 bar	14	1	12/3½	½	A	L	L
Carb Wise, chocolate peanut crunch	1 bar	23	0	10/5	1	A	L	L
Clif (average)	1 bar	43	21	4/2	5	A	A	A
EAS AdvantEdge, chocolate peanut crisp	1 bar	32	19	6/3	1	A	A	A
EAS AdvantEdge Carb Control (sugar free)	1 bar	27	1	7/5	6	A	G	G
Kudos Bar-type, whole grain, chocolate chip	1⅓ oz	20	13	5/2½	1	A	A	A

BARS (CONT.)

Food	Portion	Total Carbs (g)	Total Sugar (g)	Fat/ Sat Fat (g)	Fiber (g)	Ph 1	Ph 2	Ph 3
Luna (average)	1 bar	26	14	4/3	2	A	A	A
Pria Power Bars, chocolate peanut crunch	1 bar	16	10	3/2	0	A	A	V
Pure Protein (average)	1 bar	17	6	5/3	0	A	L	L
Slim Fast Bars (average)	1 bar	19	10	5/3	2	A	A	A
South Beach Chocolate Crisp	1 bar	26	0	6/3	5	A	G	G
South Beach Chocolate Peanut Butter	1 bar	26	<1	7/3	6	A	G	G
South Beach Cinnamon Crème	1 bar	26	<1	7/3	5	A	G	G
Sports bar, Power Bar-type, chocolate	2¼ oz	45	14	2/1½	3	A	A	A
Zone Perfect (average)	1 bar	21	16	7/4	1	A	V	L

SHAKES

Food	Portion	Total Carbs (g)	Total Sugar (g)	Fat/ Sat Fat (g)	Fiber (g)	Ph 1	Ph 2	Ph 3
Atkins Advantage Shake	11 oz	5	1	9/1½	3	G	G	G
Carb Solution Shake	8 oz	5	1	1/½	3	G	G	G
EAS AdvantEdge Carb Control	8 oz	4	0	3/½	2	G	G	G
EAS Myoplex Carb Sense	11 oz	5	0	3½/½	2	L	L	L

Food	Portion	Total Carbs (g)	Total Sugar (g)	Fat/ Sat Fat (g)	Fiber (g)	Ph 1	Ph 2	Ph 3
Keto Low Carb Shake	8 oz	9	0	9/1	7	G	G	G
Slim Fast Meal Shake	12 oz	7	2	9/1½	5	G	G	G
Slim Fast Meal Optima	11 oz	40	35	2½/½	5	A	A	A

MEATS, PROCESSED MEATS, AND MEAT SUBSTITUTES

Many beef options are appropriate for a heart-healthy diet. To select the leanest cuts, look for "round" or "loin" in the name.

Processed meats are those products which are made from meat, such as beef, chicken, or turkey, and then "processed" into a "form." These include bologna, bratwurst, hot dogs, jerky, and sausage. Most of these products contain sodium nitrate as a preservative for longer shelf life and are, as a rule, extremely high in saturated fat and sodium.

Tofu, tempeh, and other soy-based foods are all good meat substitutes. When you eat these, you also benefit from soy's cholesterol-lowering properties.

BEEF

Food	Portion	Total Carbs (g)	Total Sugar (g)	Fat/ Sat Fat (g)	Fiber (g)	Ph 1	Ph 2	Ph 3
Beef roasts								
Bottom round, braised	3 oz	0	0	6/2½	0	G	G	G
Eye round, roasted	3 oz	0	0	3½/1	0	G	G	G
Pot roast, arm, braised	3 oz	0	0	7/2½	0	G	G	G
Pot roast, blade, braised	3 oz	0	0	11/4½	0	A	A	L
Rib eye, roasted	3 oz	0	0	8/3	0	A	A	L

BEEF (CONT.)

Food	Portion	Total Carbs (g)	Total Sugar (g)	Fat/ Sat Fat (g)	Fiber (g)	Ph 1	Ph 2	Ph 3
Beef roasts (cont.)								
Shank, cross-cut, braised	3 oz	0	0	5/2	0	G	G	G
Short ribs, braised	3 oz	0	0	15/7	0	A	A	A
Sirloin tip, roasted	3 oz	0	0	7/2½	0	G	G	G
Beef steaks								
London broil, flank	3 oz	0	0	7/3	0	G	G	G
Porterhouse, broiled	3 oz	0	0	10/3½	0	G	G	G
Rib eye, broiled	3 oz	0	0	6/2½	0	A	A	L
Sirloin strip, broiled	3 oz	0	0	6/2½	0	G	G	G
T-bone, broiled	3 oz	0	0	8/3½	0	G	G	G
Tenderloin, broiled	3 oz	0	0	7/2½	0	G	G	G
Top round, panfried	3 oz	0	0	12/4	0	A	A	A
Top sirloin, broiled	3 oz	0	0	6/2	0	G	G	G
Briskets								
Corned beef, braised	3 oz	0	0	16/5	0	A	A	A
Flat half, braised	3 oz	0	0	8/3	0	A	A	A
Point half, braised	3 oz	0	0	12/4½	0	A	A	A
Whole, braised	3 oz	0	0	9/3	0	L	L	L
Cubes, stew, or kebabs, braised or grilled	3 oz	0	0	10/3½	0	L	L	L

MEATS, PROCESSED MEATS, AND MEAT SUBSTITUTES

Food	Portion	Total Carbs (g)	Total Sugar (g)	Fat/ Sat Fat (g)	Fiber (g)	Ph 1	Ph 2	Ph 3
Ground beef								
Extra-lean, baked or broiled (5% fat)	3 oz	0	0	5/2½	0	G	G	G
Lean, baked or broiled (10% fat)	3 oz	0	0	9/3½	0	L	L	L
Regular, baked or broiled (15% fat)	3 oz	0	0	12/4½	0	V	V	V

LAMB

Food	Portion	Total Carbs (g)	Total Sugar (g)	Fat/ Sat Fat (g)	Fiber (g)	Ph 1	Ph 2	Ph 3
Cubes, stew, or kebabs, braised or grilled	3 oz	0	0	6/2	0	G	G	G
Leg of lamb								
Shank half, roasted	3 oz	0	0	6/2½	0	G	G	G
Sirloin half, roasted	3 oz	0	0	9/4	0	G	G	G
Whole, roasted	3 oz	0	0	13/6	0	A	A	V
Loin chop, broiled	3 oz	0	0	7/2½	0	G	G	G
Rib, roast, crown rack of lamb, roasted	3 oz	0	0	10/4½	0	A	A	V
Rib chop, broiled	3 oz	0	0	8/4	0	L	L	L

Food	Portion	Total Carbs (g)	Total Sugar (g)	Fat/ Sat Fat (g)	Fiber (g)	Ph 1	Ph 2	Ph 3
Pork chitterlings (stewed)	1 oz	0	0	8/3	0	A	A	A
Pork chops								
Blade, braised	3 oz	0	0	11/4	0	L	L	L
Center loin, broiled	3 oz	0	0	7/2½	0	G	G	G
Sirloin, braised	3 oz	0	0	6/2	0	G	G	G
Top loin, broiled	3 oz	0	0	3½/1½	0	G	G	G
Pork cutlets								
Center slice, smoked ham, broiled or panfried	3 oz	0	0	8/3	0	L	L	L
Cutlet, braised or panfried	3 oz	0	0	8/3	0	L	L	L
Sirloin roast cutlet, braised or panfried	3 oz	0	0	8/3	0	G	G	G
Pork roasts								
Boston blade, braised	3 oz	0	0	13/4½	0	A	A	V
Center loin, roasted	3 oz	0	0	8/3	0	G	G	G
Center rib, roasted	3 oz	0	0	9/3½	0	L	L	L
Fresh ham, whole, roasted	3 oz	0	0	8/3	0	G	G	G
Half shank, roasted	3 oz	0	0	9/3	0	G	G	G
Sirloin, roasted	3 oz	0	0	7/2½	0	G	G	G
Tenderloin, roasted	3 oz	0	0	4/1½	0	G	G	G
Top loin, roasted	3 oz	0	0	6/2	0	G	G	G

Food	Portion	Total Carbs (g)	Total Sugar (g)	Fat/ Sat Fat (g)	Fiber (g)	Ph 1	Ph 2	Ph 3
Ribs								
Back ribs, full-fat, roasted	3 oz	0	0	25/9	0	A	A	A
Spareribs, country-style, lean, braised	3 oz	0	0	12/5	0	A	A	A
Spareribs, full-fat, braised	3 oz	0	0	25/9	0	A	A	A

PORK, CURED

Food	Portion	Total Carbs (g)	Total Sugar (g)	Fat/ Sat Fat (g)	Fiber (g)	Ph 1	Ph 2	Ph 3
Bacon								
Bacon bits	1 Tbsp	0	0	2/1	0	A	L	L
Breakfast strips, broiled	2 med. strips (½ ounce)	0	0	5/2	0	A	A	A
Canadian, grilled	3 oz	0	0	7/2½	0	G	G	G
Ham, cured, roasted								
Boneless, extra-lean	3 oz	0	0	4½/1½	0	G	G	G
Boneless, lean	3 oz	0	0	8/3	0	G	G	G
Canned, extra-lean	3 oz	0	0	4/1½	0	G	G	G
Canned, lean	3 oz	0	0	7/2½	0	G	G	G

VEAL

Food	Portion	Total Carbs (g)	Total Sugar (g)	Fat/ Sat Fat (g)	Fiber (g)	Ph 1	Ph 2	Ph 3
Cutlet, braised	3 oz	0	0	3/1	0	G	G	G
Ground, broiled	3 oz	0	0	6/2½	0	G	G	G

VEAL (CONT.)

Food	Portion	Total Carbs (g)	Total Sugar (g)	Fat/ Sat Fat (g)	Fiber (g)	Ph 1	Ph 2	Ph 3
Loin chop, braised	3 oz	0	0	8/2	0	G	G	G
Shank, stewed	3 oz	0	0	2½/½	0	G	G	G

PROCESSED MEATS

Food	Portion	Total Carbs (g)	Total Sugar (g)	Fat/ Sat Fat (g)	Fiber (g)	Ph 1	Ph 2	Ph 3
Hot dogs, cooked								
Beef, fat-free	1 each	7	2	0/0	0	G	G	G
Beef, light, reduced-fat	1 each	3	1	7/3	0	A	A	A
Beef, regular	1 each	3	2	16/7	0	A	A	A
Beef and pork	1 each	1	1	17/6	0	A	A	A
Chicken	1 each	0	0	12/4	0	A	A	A
Turkey and cheese	1 each	1	1	13/4½	0	A	A	A
Turkey and pork	1 each	1	1	13/4½	0	A	A	A
Sandwich meats								
Bologna, beef	2 oz	0	0	16/7	0	A	A	A
Bologna, beef and pork	2 oz	3	1	13/5	0	A	A	A
Bologna, chicken	2 oz	1	0	13/3½	0	A	A	A
Bologna, lebanon	2 oz	0	0	6/1½	0	A	A	A
Bologna, pork	2 oz	0	0	11/4	0	A	A	A
Bologna, turkey	2 oz	0	0	12/3	0	A	A	A
Chicken roll (light meat)	2 oz	0	0	1½/0	0	L	L	L
Corned beef	2 oz	0	0	2½/1½	0	A	A	L
Dried beef (not jerky)	2 oz	2	1	1/½	0	L	L	L

Food	Portion	Total Carbs (g)	Total Sugar (g)	Fat/ Sat Fat (g)	Fiber (g)	Ph 1	Ph 2	Ph 3
Ham, boiled, deli thin	2 oz	1	1	½/0	0	G	G	G
Ham, chopped	2 oz	2	0	6/2	0	G	G	G
Ham, honey loaf	2 oz	2	2	2/½	0	A	A	A
Ham, turkey	2 oz	2	2	3/1	0	G	G	G
Pastrami, beef	2 oz	1	1	3½/1½	0	L	L	L
Pastrami, turkey	2 oz	1	0	2½/1	0	G	G	G
Pickle and pimiento loaf	2 oz	5	2	9/3	0	A	A	A
Salami, beef	2 oz	1	1	13/6	0	A	A	A
Salami, genoa	2 oz	1	0	19/7	0	A	A	A
Salami, hard	2 oz	1	0	16/6	0	A	A	A
Turkey breast, smoked	2 oz	3	1	1½/½	0	G	G	G
Turkey roll (light meat)	2 oz	1	0	2/½	0	L	L	L
Turkey bacon (2 slices)	1 oz	0	0	5/2	0	L	G	G
Turkey sausage	2 oz.	3	2	5/2	0	L	G	G
Sausages, cooked								
Bratwurst (pork)	2 oz	1	0	11/4	0	A	A	A
Italian, sweet	2 oz	1	0	5/2	0	A	A	A
Kielbasa (pork/beef)	2 oz	1	0	15/6	0	A	A	A
Knockwurst (beef)	2 oz	1	0	16/7	0	A	A	A
Pork, patty	2 oz	0	0	16/5	0	A	A	A
Summer (beef)	2 oz	1	1	15/7	0	A	A	A
Turkey, patty	2 oz	0	0	7/2	0	G	G	G

MEAT SUBSTITUTES

Food	Portion	Total Carbs (g)	Total Sugar (g)	Fat/ Sat Fat (g)	Fiber (g)	Ph 1	Ph 2	Ph 3
Burgers and hot dogs								
Black bean burger	1 each	15	2	1/0	3	G	G	G
Hot dog, Tofu Pup, frozen	1 each	28	0	2½/1	0	G	G	G
Seitan (wheat gluten), refrigerated, ready to serve (oriental)	4 oz	10	0	2/0	0	G	G	G
Tempeh soy burger (BBQ)	1 each	11	3	3½/1½	0	G	G	G
Veggie burger (Garden burger)	1 each	10	1	4/½	4	G	G	G
Tempeh (soybean)								
Fakin' Bacon, tempeh strips	2 med. strips (1 oz)	3	0	1/0	0	G	G	G
Five grain	⅓ package	15	2	4/½	4	G	G	G
Original, plain	⅓ package	13	2	5/½	5	G	G	G
Wild rice	⅓ package	17	1	2½/½	5	G	G	G
Tofu (soybean)								
Baked and seasoned, refrigerated, ready to serve	3 oz	5	0	9/1½	2	L	G	G
Raw, firm, refrigerated	3 oz	4	0	7/1	2	G	G	G
Silken, refrigerated	3 oz	2	1	1½/0	0	G	G	G

Dairy products are an excellent source of calcium and protein and make for great snacks. But whole-milk dairy products, such as butter, cheese, milk, cream, and ice cream contain high amounts of saturated fat. When selecting dairy products, look for non-fat or low-fat varieties of milk or plain yogurt or yogurt sweetened with aspartame. These products contain the milk sugar lactose, which has a moderated glycemic index lower than other simple sugars. Also look for low-fat soy milk and soy drinks, which contain more protein and less fat than cow's milk.

CREAMS AND CREAMERS

Food	Portion	Total Carbs (g)	Total Sugar (g)	Fat/ Sat Fat (g)	Fiber (g)	Ph 1	Ph 2	Ph 3
Cream								
Half & half	2 Tbsp	1	0	3/2	0	V	V	V
Light	2 Tbsp	1	0	6/3½	0	L	L	L
Medium	2 Tbsp	1	0	7/4½	0	V	V	V
Creamers, nondairy								
Liquid, refrigerated, fat-free	2 Tbsp	4	0	0/0	0	G	G	G
Liquid, refrigerated, flavored, sweetened	2 Tbsp	14	12	3/0	0	A	A	A
Liquid, refrigerated, light	2 Tbsp	1	0	1½/½	0	G	G	G
Liquid, refrigerated, regular, plain	2 Tbsp	4	1	2½/½	0	L	L	L
Powdered, original	1 tsp	1	0	½/½	0	G	G	G

CREAMS AND CREAMERS (CONT.)

MILK, MILK PRODUCTS, AND MILK SUBSTITUTES

Food	Portion	Total Carbs (g)	Total Sugar (g)	Fat/ Sat Fat (g)	Fiber (g)	Ph 1	Ph 2	Ph 3
Sour cream								
Fat-free	2 Tbsp	5	2	0/0	0	G	G	G
Imitation, plain	2 Tbsp	2	2	6/5	0	L	L	L
Nondairy, substitute, plain	2 Tbsp	3	0	3/0	0	G	G	G
Reduced-fat	2 Tbsp	1	0	3½/2	0	G	G	G
Regular, plain	2 Tbsp	1	0	6/4	0	A	A	V
Toppings, whipped								
Dessert cream topping, frozen, extra-creamy	2 Tbsp	2	2	2/2	0	V	V	V
Dessert cream topping, frozen, light	2 Tbsp	2	1	1/1	0	G	G	G
Dessert cream topping, frozen, nondairy	2 Tbsp	2	1	2/2	0	G	G	G
Whipped cream, pressurized	2 Tbsp	1	0	1½/1	0	L	L	L
Whipping cream								
Heavy, liquid	1 Tbsp	1	1	6/3½	0	A	A	V
Heavy, whipped	¼ cup	1	1	11/7	0	A	A	V
Heavy, whipped, from ½ cup liquid	1 cup	3	3	44/27	0	A	A	V
Light, liquid	1 Tbsp	1	1	4½/3	0	A	A	V
Light, whipped	¼ cup	1	1	9/6	0	A	A	V
Light, whipped, from ½ cup liquid	1 cup	4	4	37/23	0	A	A	V

MILK AND NONDAIRY MILKS

Food	Portion	Total Carbs (g)	Total Sugar (g)	Fat/ Sat Fat (g)	Fiber (g)	Ph 1	Ph 2	Ph 3
Buttermilk, low-fat, 1%	8 fl oz	13	12	2½/1½	0	G	G	G
Buttermilk, reduced-fat, 2%	8 fl oz	12	12	5/2	0	L	L	L
Chocolate Milk								
Low-fat, 1%	8 fl oz	26	22	3/1½	0	A	A	A
Reduced-fat, 2%	8 fl oz	26	25	5/3	1	A	A	A
Whole milk	8 fl oz	26	24	8/5	2	A	A	A
Cow's milk								
Fat-free/skim	8 fl oz	12	12	0/0	0	G	G	G
Low-fat/light, 1%	8 fl oz	12	12	2½/1½	0	G	G	G
Protein-fortified, 1%	8 fl oz	14	11	3/2	0	A	A	A
Reduced-fat, 2%	8 fl oz	13	13	5/3	0	A	V	L
Whole, 3½%	8 fl oz	11	11	8/4½	0	A	V	L
Eggnog, reduced-fat	4 fl oz	20	19	4½/2½	0	A	A	V
Eggnog, regular	4 fl oz	25	24	9/5	0	A	A	A
Low-lactose								
Fat-free	8 fl oz	12	12	0/0	0	G	G	G
Low-fat, 1%	8 fl oz	13	12	2½/1½	0	G	G	G
Reduced-fat, 2%	8 fl oz	13	12	5/3	0	A	V	L
Other milks and kefir								
Acidophilus milk, low-fat, 1%	8 fl oz	12	12	3/1½	0	G	G	G
Acidophilus milk, reduced-fat, 2%	8 fl oz	12	12	5/3	0	A	V	L

MILK AND NONDAIRY MILKS (CONT.)

Food	Portion	Total Carbs (g)	Total Sugar (g)	Fat/ Sat Fat (g)	Fiber (g)	Ph 1	Ph 2	Ph 3
Other milks and kefir (cont.)								
Goat's milk, low-fat	8 fl oz	9	9	3/1	0	G	G	G
Goat's milk, whole	8 fl oz	11	11	10/7	0	A	A	V
Kefir, plain (non fat)	8 fl oz	11	11	0/0	0	G	G	G
Canned milk								
Evaporated, fat-free	2 Tbsp	4	4	0/0	0	G	G	G
Evaporated, low-fat	2 Tbsp	3	3	½/½	0	G	G	G
Evaporated, whole	2 Tbsp	3	3	2½/1½	0	A	A	A
Sweetened condensed, fat-free	2 Tbsp	24	24	0/0	0	A	A	A
Sweetened condensed, low-fat	2 Tbsp	23	23	1½/1	0	A	A	A
Sweetened condensed, regular	2 Tbsp	21	21	3½/2	0	A	A	A
Dry milk								
Buttermilk	1 oz	14	14	2/1	0	G	G	G
Nonfat	1 oz	15	15	0/0	0	G	G	G
Whole milk	1 oz	11	11	8/4½	0	A	A	V

SOY MILK

Food	Portion	Total Carbs (g)	Total Sugar (g)	Fat/ Sat Fat (g)	Fiber (g)	Ph 1	Ph 2	Ph 3
Chocolate, refrigerated	8 fl oz	23	19	4/0	3	A	A	V
Plain, refrigerated	8 fl oz	8	4	4/0	0	G	G	G
Soy milk creamer, refrigerated	2 Tbsp	6	6	2/0	0	G	G	G
Unsweetened, refrigerated	8 fl oz	5	1	4/½	1	G	G	G
Vanilla, refrigerated	8 fl oz	10	7	4/½	1	A	V	L

YOGURTS

Food	Portion	Total Carbs (g)	Total Sugar (g)	Fat/ Sat Fat (g)	Fiber (g)	Ph 1	Ph 2	Ph 3
Fruited								
Fat-free, sweetened w/sugar	8 oz	22	17	0/0	0	A	A	A
Light, fat-free, artificially sweetened	8 oz	18	17	0/0	1	A	L	L
Low-fat, drinkable	8 oz	36	34	3/2½	0	A	A	A
Low-fat, sweetened w/sugar	8 oz	43	37	2/1½	0	A	A	A
Whole milk, sweetened w/sugar	8 oz	38	31	6/3	1	A	A	A
Plain								
Fat-free	8 oz	18	12	0/0	0	G	G	G
Low-fat	8 oz	16	16	4/2½	0	G	G	G
Whole milk	8 oz	11	11	7/5	0	A	A	V

Food	Portion	Total Carbs (g)	Total Sugar (g)	Fat/ Sat Fat (g)	Fiber (g)	Ph 1	Ph 2	Ph 3
Soy yogurt, fruited, sweetened w/evaporated cane juice	8 oz	38	28	3/0	1	A	A	A
Soy yogurt, plain	8 oz	22	12	3/0	1	G	G	G

NUTS, NUT BUTTERS, AND SEEDS

News of the positive health benefits of nuts continues to accumulate. Nuts are a great source of good fats and protein, and consumption of nuts has been associated with decreased risks of heart attacks. Almonds, Brazil nuts, peanuts, pistachios, and many other nuts are all good choices. Walnuts are particularly rich in omega=3's. Natural nut butters appear to have the same health benefits as whole nuts, but it is important to read the labels to make sure that hydrogenated oils are not listed as ingredients. Smuckers, for example, has a natural peanut butter made without trans fats that is a good choice. But while nuts are a great source of good fats, they're also very easy to overeat, which can impede weight loss, so be mindful of how many you're consuming.

NUTS

Food	Portion	Total Carbs (g)	Total Sugar (g)	Fat/ Sat Fat (g)	Fiber (g)	Ph 1	Ph 2	Ph 3
Almonds, raw or roasted	1 oz	7	2	14/1	3	G	G	G
Brazil nuts, raw	1 oz	4	1	19/4½	2	G	G	G
Cashews, roasted	1 oz	10	2	14/2½	1	G	G	G
Filberts (hazelnuts), roasted	1 oz	5	1	17/1½	3	G	G	G
Macadamias, raw	1 oz	5	2	20/1½	2	G	G	G
Peanuts, roasted	1 oz	6	1	14/2	2	G	G	G
Pecans, dried	1 oz	5	1	20/2	3	G	G	G

Food	Portion	Total Carbs (g)	Total Sugar (g)	Fat/ Sat Fat (g)	Fiber (g)	Ph 1	Ph 2	Ph 3
Pine nuts, dried	1 oz	4	1	19/1½	1	G	G	G
Pistachios, shelled	1 oz	8	2	13/1½	3	G	G	G
Soy nuts, roasted	1 oz	9	0	7/1	5	G	G	G
Walnuts, English, dried	1 oz	4	1	18/1½	2	G	G	G

NUT BUTTERS

Food	Portion	Total Carbs (g)	Total Sugar (g)	Fat/ Sat Fat (g)	Fiber (g)	Ph 1	Ph 2	Ph 3
Almond butter	1 Tbsp	3	2	9/1	0	G	G	G
Cashew butter	1 Tbsp	5	1	7/1½	0	G	G	G
Hazelnut butter	1 Tbsp	3	2	10/½	1	G	G	G
Peanut butter, reduced-fat	1 Tbsp	8	3	6/1½	1	V	V	V
Peanut butter, w/no added sugar, freshly ground	1 Tbsp	4	1	8/1	1	G	G	G
Pistachio butter	1 Tbsp	5	2	9/1	2	G	G	G
Sesame seed paste (tahini)	1 Tbsp	2	0	9/1	0	G	G	G
Soy nut butter	1 Tbsp	6	1	6/1	1	G	G	G

SEEDS

Food	Portion	Total Carbs (g)	Total Sugar (g)	Fat/ Sat Fat (g)	Fiber (g)	Ph 1	Ph 2	Ph 3
Flaxseed	1 Tbsp	3	0	3½/0	3	G	G	G
Poppy	1 Tbsp	2	1	4/0	0	G	G	G
Pumpkin (pepitas)	1 Tbsp	2	0	1/0	0	G	G	G
Sesame	1 Tbsp	2	0	4½/½	1	G	G	G
Sunflower	1 Tbsp	2	0	4½/0	0	G	G	G

PASTA AND PASTA DISHES

Whole wheat pasta is the preferred type of pasta on the South Beach Diet. We recommended that you boil the pasta until just tender or "al dente." Also, to reduce portion size, try eating pasta as a side dish to your fish or chicken, rather than a stand-alone entrée.

Enjoy your pasta with a low-sugar tomato sauce. Research shows that lycopene in tomatoes can be more efficiently absorbed when processed into tomato sauces or tomato paste. This is important because lycopene has been shown to help prevent prostate cancer.

PASTA, COOKED

Food	Portion	Total Carbs (g)	Total Sugar (g)	Fat/ Sat Fat (g)	Fiber (g)	Ph 1	Ph 2	Ph 3
Capellini, semolina	1 cup	43	2	1/0	2	A	V	L
Corn pasta, gluten-free	1 cup	39	3	1/0	1	A	A	A
Egg noodle, homemade, plain, spinach, or tomato	1 cup	40	1	2/0	2	A	V	L
Fettuccine, egg noodle, spinach	1 cup	40	2	2/1	2	A	V	L
Linguine, semolina	1 cup	42	1	1/0	2	A	V	L
Macaroni, semolina	1 cup	39	2	1/0	2	A	V	L
Macaroni, whole wheat	1 cup	38	1	1/0	4	A	G	G
Rice pasta, brown	1 cup	39	1	2/0	1	A	A	V
Spaghetti, semolina	1 cup	41	1	1/0	2	A	V	L
Spaghetti, whole wheat	1 cup	39	1	1/0	6	A	G	G
Vermicelli, semolina	1 cup	42	2	1/0	2	A	V	L

PASTA DISHES, PREPARED WITH SEMOLINA PASTA

Food	Portion	Total Carbs (g)	Total Sugar (g)	Fat/ Sat Fat (g)	Fiber (g)	Ph 1	Ph 2	Ph 3
Gnocchi, potato dumpling	1 cup	75	11	3/1½	4	A	A	V
Lasagna, w/meat sauce, homemade	1 cup	38	6	16/8	3	A	A	V
Lasagna, w/spinach, vegetarian, homemade	1 cup	41	7	10/6	5	A	V	L
Macaroni and cheese, baked, homemade	1 cup	30	6	14/9	1	A	A	V
Macaroni and cheese, prepared from box	1 cup	49	8	18/4½	1	A	A	A
Meat ravioli, w/meat sauce	1 cup	36	7	17/6	3	A	A	V
Meat ravioli, w/tomato sauce	1 cup	38	10	18/6	3	A	A	V
Pasta primavera	1 cup	51	7	4/1	5	A	V	L
Spaghetti								
W/marinara sauce	1 cup	32	6	3/½	4	A	V	L
W/meatballs and marinara sauce	1 cup	29	6	10/2	8	A	V	L
W/red clam sauce	1 cup	41	8	8/1	3	A	V	L
W/white clam sauce	1 cup	43	5	20/2½	2	A	A	V
Tortellini, cheese, w/tomato sauce	1 cup	43	2	10/4	3	A	A	V

PICKLES, PEPPERS, AND RELISH

Pickles, peppers, and relishes are all okay as long as they are not the sweet-ened versions.

Food	Portion	Total Carbs (g)	Total Sugar (g)	Fat/ Sat Fat (g)	Fiber (g)	Ph 1	Ph 2	Ph 3
Bread and butter pickles, sweetened	3 pieces	5	5	0/0	0	A	A	A
Dill pickle	1 large	5	2	0/0	2	L	L	L
Gherkin, sweet	1 medium	5	5	0/0	1	A	A	A
Green chiles, chopped	2 Tbsp	2	1	0/0	0	G	G	G
Jalapeño peppers, pickled	2 whole	2	1	0/0	0	G	G	G
Peppers, roasted, whole, red or yellow, jarred	½ of whole	2	1	2/0	0	G	G	G
Sauerkraut, drained	½ cup	3	1	0/0	2	G	G	G
Sweet gherkin pickle relish, sweetened	1 Tbsp	5	1	0/0	0	A	V	V

PIZZA

If pizza is among your favorite treats, have a thin-crust pizza with tomato sauce, reduced-fat cheese, and/or vegetables. Thick-crust pizzas, as well as those made on French bread, are trouble. Also steer clear of high saturated fat toppings, such as mixed cheeses, pepperoni, and sausage.

FRENCH BREAD PIZZA, FROZEN

Food	Portion	Total Carbs (g)	Total Sugar (g)	Fat/ Sat Fat (g)	Fiber (g)	Ph 1	Ph 2	Ph 3
Deluxe cheese	1 serving	45	2	21/6	4	A	A	A
Pepperoni	1 serving	43	3	17/6	3	A	A	A

Food	Portion	Total Carbs (g)	Total Sugar (g)	Fat/ Sat Fat (g)	Fiber (g)	Ph 1	Ph 2	Ph 3
Sausage	1 serving	48	5	18/7	3	A	A	A
White cheese	1 serving	45	2	25/7	3	A	A	A

PIZZA, TRADITIONAL

Food	Portion	Total Carbs (g)	Total Sugar (g)	Fat/ Sat Fat (g)	Fiber (g)	Ph 1	Ph 2	Ph 3
Personal Pan Pizza (1 whole)								
Beef	10 oz	71	2	35/14	4	A	A	A
Cheese	9¼ oz	71	3	28/12	4	A	A	A
Ham	9 oz	70	2	24/8	4	A	A	A
Italian sausage	10¼ oz	71	2	39/16	5	A	A	A
Pepperoni	9 oz	70	2	28/12	4	A	A	A
Pork	9 oz	71	2	34/13	4	A	A	A
12" Hand-Tossed Pizza								
Cheese	3½ oz slice	30	5	8/4½	2	A	A	V
Pepperoni	3½ oz slice	30	7	10/4½	1	A	A	A
Sausage	4 oz slice	30	7	13/6	2	A	A	A
Vegetable	4½ oz slice	29	8	6/3	2	A	A	V
12" Pan Pizza								
Cheese	4 oz slice	29	6	13/5	1	A	A	V
Pepperoni	4½ oz slice	29	6	15/5	2	A	A	A
Sausage	4½ oz slice	29	6	12/4	2	A	A	A
Vegetable	4½ oz slice	29	6	17/6	2	A	A	V
12" Thin Crust Pizza								
Cheese	3 oz slice	21	4	8/4½	1	A	V	V
Pepperoni	3 oz slice	21	1	10/4½	1	A	A	A
Sausage	3½ oz slice	21	5	13/6	2	A	A	A

PIZZA, TRADITIONAL (CONT.)

Food	Portion	Total Carbs (g)	Total Sugar (g)	Fat/ Sat Fat (g)	Fiber (g)	Ph 1	Ph 2	Ph 3
Frozen Pizza								
South Beach Diet Four Cheese	1 whole	33	6	9/4	14	A	G	G
South Beach Diet Pepperoni	1 whole	33	6	10/4	14	A	G	G
South Beach Diet Chicken Vegetable	1 whole	34	6	8/3½	14	A	G	G
Whole Wheat Pizza								
Four cheese	2¾ oz slice	19	2	7/3	2	A	V	L
Mushroom and spinach	2¾ oz slice	21	3	4/2	2	A	L	L
Vegetarian	2¾ oz slice	17	3	4/2	2	A	L	L

POULTRY

When it comes to chicken, bake, broil, grill, roast, or sauté, but do not fry. Select the chicken breast, which has far less saturated fat than the leg, thigh, and wing, and remove the skin before eating. Duck and goose are higher in saturated fat than chicken and should not be eaten often.

CHICKEN (AN AVERAGE OF LIGHT AND DARK MEAT)

Food	Portion	Total Carbs (g)	Total Sugar (g)	Fat/ Sat Fat (g)	Fiber (g)	Ph 1	Ph 2	Ph 3
Fried, batter-dipped	4 oz	11	0	20/5	0	A	A	A
Fried, flour-coated	4 oz	4	0	17/5	0	A	A	A
Roasted, w/skin	4 oz	0	0	15/4½	0	V	V	V
Roasted, without skin	4 oz	0	0	8/2½	0	G	G	G
Stewed, w/skin	4 oz	0	0	14/4	0	V	V	V
Stewed, without skin	4 oz	0	0	8/2	0	G	G	G

CHICKEN, ORGAN MEATS, SIMMERED

Food	Portion	Total Carbs (g)	Total Sugar (g)	Fat/ Sat Fat (g)	Fiber (g)	Ph 1	Ph 2	Ph 3
Giblets	½ cup	1	0	4/1½	0	A	A	A
Gizzard	½ cup	0	0	3/0	0	A	A	V
Heart	½ cup	0	0	6/1½	0	A	A	A
Liver	½ cup	1	0	4/1½	0	A	A	A

CHICKEN, PARTS, BROILERS OR FRYERS

Food	Portion	Total Carbs (g)	Total Sugar (g)	Fat/ Sat Fat (g)	Fiber (g)	Ph 1	Ph 2	Ph 3
Breast (½ breast)								
Fried, batter-dipped, w/skin	5 oz	12	0	19/5	0	A	A	A
Fried, flour-coated, w/skin	3½ oz	2	0	9/2½	0	A	A	A
Roasted, w/skin (from 5 oz raw)	3½ oz	0	0	8/2	0	V	V	V
Roasted, without skin (from 4¼ oz raw)	3 oz	0	0	3/1	0	G	G	G
Stewed, w/skin	3½ oz	0	0	7/2	0	V	V	V
Stewed, without skin	3 oz	0	0	3/½	0	G	G	G
Drumstick								
Fried, batter-dipped, w/skin	2½ oz	6	0	11/3	0	A	A	A
Fried, flour-coated, w/skin	1¾ oz	1	0	7/2	0	A	A	A
Roasted, w/skin	2 oz	0	0	6/1½	0	V	V	V
Roasted, without skin	1½ oz	0	0	2½/½	0	L	L	L

CHICKEN, PARTS, BROILERS OR FRYERS (CONT.)

Food	Portion	Total Carbs (g)	Total Sugar (g)	Fat/ Sat Fat (g)	Fiber (g)	Ph 1	Ph 2	Ph 3
Drumstick (cont.)								
Stewed, w/skin	2 oz	0	0	6/1½	0	V	V	V
Stewed, without skin	1½ oz	0	0	3/½	0	L	L	L
Thigh								
Fried, batter-dipped, w/skin	3 oz	8	0	14/4	0	A	A	A
Fried, flour-coated, w/skin	2¼ oz	2	0	10/2½	0	A	A	A
Roasted, w/skin (from 4 oz raw w/bone)	2½ oz	0	0	11/3	0	V	V	V
Roasted, without skin (from 4 oz raw w/bone)	2 oz	0	0	6/1½	0	L	L	L
Stewed, w/skin	2½ oz	0	0	10/3	0	V	V	V
Stewed, without skin	2 oz	0	0	6/1½	0	L	L	L
Wing								
Fried, batter-dipped, w/skin	1¾ oz	5	0	11/3	0	A	A	A
Fried, flour-coated, w/skin	1 oz	1	0	6/1½	0	A	A	A
Roasted, w/skin (from 3 oz raw w/bone)	1¼ oz	0	0	7/2	0	V	V	V
Roasted, without skin (from 2½ oz raw w/bone)	¾ oz	0	0	2/0	0	L	L	L

CHICKEN, ROASTERS

Food	Portion	Total Carbs (g)	Total Sugar (g)	Fat/ Sat Fat (g)	Fiber (g)	Ph 1	Ph 2	Ph 3
Dark meat, without skin, roasted	3 oz	0	0	7/2	0	L	L	L
Light and dark meat (an average), roasted w/skin	4 oz	0	0	15/4	0	V	V	V
Light and dark meat (an average), roasted without skin	4 oz	0	0	8/2	0	L	L	L
Light meat, without skin, roasted	3 oz	0	0	4/1	0	G	G	G

CHICKEN, STEWING

Food	Portion	Total Carbs (g)	Total Sugar (g)	Fat/ Sat Fat (g)	Fiber (g)	Ph 1	Ph 2	Ph 3
Dark meat, without skin (stewed)	3 oz	0	0	13/3½	0	L	L	L
Light and dark meat, (an average), w/skin	4 oz	0	0	21/6	0	V	V	V
Light and dark meat, (an average), without skin	4 oz	0	0	13/3½	0	L	L	L
Light meat, without skin	3 oz	0	0	7/1½	0	G	G	G

TURKEY

Food	Portion	Total Carbs (g)	Total Sugar (g)	Fat/ Sat Fat (g)	Fiber (g)	Ph 1	Ph 2	Ph 3
Dark meat, w/skin	3½ oz	0	0	11/3½	0	V	V	V
Dark meat, without skin	3 oz	0	0	6/2	0	L	L	L

TURKEY (CONT.)

Food	Portion	Total Carbs (g)	Total Sugar (g)	Fat/ Sat Fat (g)	Fiber (g)	Ph 1	Ph 2	Ph 3
Light meat, w/skin	3½ oz	0	0	8/2½	0	L	L	L
Light meat, without skin	3 oz	0	0	2½/1	0	G	G	G
Turkey parts								
Back, roasted, w/skin	4½ oz	0	0	18/5	0	V	V	V
Back, roasted, without skin	3½ oz	0	0	6/2	0	L	L	L
Breast meat, , roasted, w/skin	4¼ oz	0	0	9/2½	0	V	V	V
Breast meat, roasted, without skin	3 oz	0	0	½/0	0	G	G	G
Giblets, simmered	1 cup	0	0	17/6	0	A	A	A
Leg (thigh and drumstick), roasted, w/skin	8¼ oz	0	0	23/7	0	V	V	V
Leg (thigh and drumstick), roasted, without skin	7½ oz	0	0	8/2½	0	L	L	L
Neck, simmered, w/bone without skin	9 oz	0	0	19/6	0	V	V	V
Wing, roasted, w/skin	3 oz	0	0	11/3	0	V	V	V
Wing, roasted, without skin	2 oz	0	0	2/½	0	L	L	L

CAPON, CORNISH HEN, DUCK, AND GOOSE

Food	Portion	Total Carbs (g)	Total Sugar (g)	Fat/ Sat Fat (g)	Fiber (g)	Ph 1	Ph 2	Ph 3
Capon, roasted, w/skin	4 oz	0	0	13/3½	0	V	V	V
Cornish hen, roasted						G	G	G
Dark meat, w/skin	3 oz	0	0	11/5	0	V	V	V
Dark meat, without skin	3 oz	0	0	7/3	0	L	L	L
Light meat, w/skin	3 oz	0	0	8/2½	0	L	L	L
Light meat, without skin	3 oz	0	0	3/1½	0	G	G	G
Duck, roasted, w/skin	3 oz	0	0	33/11	0	A	A	A
Duck, roasted, without skin	3 oz	0	0	10/3½	0	V	V	V
Goose, roasted, w/skin	3 oz	0	0	19/6	0	A	A	A
Goose, roasted, without skin	3 oz	0	0	1¼	0	V	V	V

SALADS AND SALAD DRESSINGS

Prepared salads, such as tuna or egg, can be an occasional part of your diet, but the best salads are those with mixed greens and a flavorful vinaigrette dressing.

SALADS

Food	Portion	Total Carbs (g)	Total Sugar (g)	Fat/ Sat Fat (g)	Fiber (g)	Ph 1	Ph 2	Ph 3
Antipasto	1 cup	5	1	10/5	2	A	A	A
Bean salad	1 cup	23	4	8/1	8	G	G	G

SALADS (CONT.)

Food	Portion	Total Carbs (g)	Total Sugar (g)	Fat/ Sat Fat (g)	Fiber (g)	Ph 1	Ph 2	Ph 3
Caesar salad, w/dressing	1 cup	15	2	15/3	2	G	G	G
Chef salad, w/turkey, ham, and cheese, no dressing	1 cup	3	0	11/5	1	L	L	L
Coleslaw, traditional, sweetened	½ cup	9	5	7/1	1	A	L	L
Cucumber salad, marinated in vinaigrette	½ cup	6	5	10/0	0	G	G	G
Egg salad	½ cup	1	1	28/5	0	G	G	G
Fresh fruit salad	1 cup	25	22	½/0	3	A	L	G
Greek salad, w/olives and feta cheese	1 cup	42	8	12/3	5	G	G	G
Grilled chicken salad	½ cup	13	9	10/3	3	G	G	G
Macaroni salad, traditional, w/egg	1 cup	29	5	37/4	2	A	A	A
Pasta salad, w/Italian vinaigrette	1 cup	33	5	16/3	1	A	A	V
Potato salad, traditional, w/egg	1 cup	33	9	15/3	6	A	A	A
Shrimp salad	½ cup	3	2	8/1½	0	G	G	G
Tabbouleh salad	½ cup	8	1	8/1	2	A	G	G
Tomato salad, w/part skim mozzarella	1 cup	5	2	12/7	0	G	G	G
Tortellini salad, w/pesto	1 cup	38	6	20/6	3	A	A	A

Food	Portion	Total Carbs (g)	Total Sugar (g)	Fat/ Sat Fat (g)	Fiber (g)	Ph 1	Ph 2	Ph 3
Tossed green salad	1 cup	5	2	0/0	2	G	G	G
Tuna salad, traditional, w/egg	½ cup	17	5	8/1½	3	G	G	G
Waldorf salad	1 cup	12	6	41/4½	3	A	A	V

SALAD DRESSINGS

Salad dressings can be land mines for many dieters because of hidden sugars and fats. However, as evidenced below, it is possible to find brands on the shelves that fit in with the nutritional principles of the South Beach Diet. Make sure to read labels carefully.

Food	Portion	Total Carbs (g)	Total Sugar (g)	Fat/ Sat Fat (g)	Fiber (g)	Ph 1	Ph 2	Ph 3
Blue cheese, reduced-fat	2 Tbsp	2	1	7/1½	0	L	L	L
Blue cheese, regular	2 Tbsp	1	0	16/2	0	L	L	L
Caesar, reduced-fat	2 Tbsp	6	5	2/0	0	L	L	L
Caesar, regular	2 Tbsp	2	2	12/2½	0	G	G	G
French								
Fat-free	2 Tbsp	11	7	0/0	0	A	A	A
Reduced-fat	2 Tbsp	6	5	3/0	0	V	V	V
Regular	2 Tbsp	5	5	14/2	0	L	L	L
Italian								
Fat-free	2 Tbsp	4	3	0/0	0	A	A	A
Reduced-fat	2 Tbsp	3	2	9/1	0	L	L	L
Regular	2 Tbsp	3	3	14/2	0	G	G	G

SALAD DRESSINGS (CONT.)

Food	Portion	Total Carbs (g)	Total Sugar (g)	Fat/ Sat Fat (g)	Fiber (g)	Ph 1	Ph 2	Ph 3
Ranch								
Fat-free	2 Tbsp	11	2	0/0	0	A	A	A
Reduced-fat	2 Tbsp	4	1	9/1½	0	L	L	L
Regular	2 Tbsp	1	1	16/2½	0	G	G	G
Russian								
Fat-free	2 Tbsp	9	5	0/0	0	A	A	A
Reduced-fat	2 Tbsp	6	4	5/1	0	L	L	L
Regular	2 Tbsp	3	3	10/1½	0	G	G	G
Thousand Island								
Fat-free	2 Tbsp	9	5	0/0	1	A	A	A
Reduced-fat	2 Tbsp	7	5	5/1	0	L	L	L
Regular	2 Tbsp	5	4	10/1½	0	G	G	G
Vinaigrette, balsamic, fat-free	2 Tbsp	6	5	0/0	0	A	A	A
Vinaigrette, balsamic, regular	2 Tbsp	4	3	14/2	0	G	G	G

A first course of soup will not only soothe your spirits, it will satisfy your appetite. Research shows that people given a first course of tomato soup ate less during subsequent courses. Good choices also include vegetable soups, such as bean, gazpacho, and lentil, which are all packed with good carbs and fiber.

Avoid cream-type soups in restaurants because they are usually made with saturated fat-laden heavy cream or whole milk. At home, make cream-type soups with water. When ordering French onion soup you might want to order it without the French bread topping.

Food	Portion	Total Carbs (g)	Total Sugar (g)	Fat/ Sat Fat (g)	Fiber (g)	Ph 1	Ph 2	Ph 3
Barley mushroom	1 cup	12	4	2½/0	1	A	G	G
Beef barley	1 cup	16	2	2/0	3	A	G	G
Beef vegetable	1 cup	17	3	2/0	1	A	G	G
Black bean	1 cup	19	2	2/0	4	G	G	G
Bouillabaisse	1 cup	6	2	9/2½	2	G	G	G
Chicken noodle	1 cup	18	1	6/1½	4	A	A	L
Chicken rice	1 cup	17	1	2/1	2	A	A	L
Clam chowder								
Manhattan, red	1 cup	12	1	2/0	1	A	V	V
New England, reduced-fat	1 cup	17	2	3/½	1	A	A	V
New England, white	1 cup	20	3	10/2½	1	A	A	A
Corn chowder, creamy	1 cup	18	4	15/3	2	A	A	A
Cream soups								
Cream of broccoli, made w/water	1 cup	17	5	3/0	2	A	G	G
Cream of chicken, made w/water	1 cup	13	3	5/3½	0	A	G	G

SOUPS (CONT.)

Food	Portion	Total Carbs (g)	Total Sugar (g)	Fat/ Sat Fat (g)	Fiber (g)	Ph 1	Ph 2	Ph 3
Cream soups (cont.)								
Cream of mushroom, made w/milk	1 cup	15	6	13/3	0	A	A	A
Cream of potato, made w/milk	1 cup	17	2	6/4	0	A	A	A
French onion soup	1 cup	22	10	4/1	2	A	L	L
Fish chowder	1 cup	18	5	6/1	0	A	L	L
Gazpacho	1 cup	4	2	0/0	0	G	G	G
Lentil	1 cup	20	2	1/0	6	G	G	G
Lentil w/ham	1 cup	20	2	3/1	6	G	G	G
Lobster bisque	1 cup	13	10	13/4	0	A	A	A
Minestrone	1 cup	20	3	3/0	5	A	L	G
Miso broth	1 cup	5	0	1½/0	0	G	G	G
Split pea	1 cup	25	4	3/1	5	A	L	L
Tomato	1 cup	17	6	2/0	0	G	G	G
Vegetable	1 cup	15	3	2/½	2	A	L	G
Vegetable, w/turkey	1 cup	9	3	3/1	0	A	L	G
Vichyssoise	1 cup	17	2	6/4	0	A	A	A

Naturally occurring sugars are those found in foods like milk products (lactose) and fruits (fructose). Refined sugars include honey, maple syrup, and table sugar. Most sugars have a low to moderate ranking on the glycemic index. Table sugar (sucrose) has a moderate ranking and can be included as part of an occasional treat or as an ingredient in baking on Phase 3.

However, sugar is the number one additive to our food supply. The typical person eats approximately 33 teaspoons of added sugar a day. Some high fructose corn syrup will be added even to products using sugar substitutes. Read and compare labels and choose wisely.

CANE SUGAR

Food	Portion	Total Carbs (g)	Total Sugar (g)	Fat/ Sat Fat (g)	Fiber (g)	Ph 1	Ph 2	Ph 3
Brown sugar	1 tsp	4	4	0/0	0	A	L	V
Raw sugar, turbinado	1 tsp	4	4	0/0	0	A	V	L
White sugar, granulated	1 tsp	4	4	0/0	0	A	V	L

JAMS, JELLIES, AND FRUIT SPREADS

Food	Portion	Total Carbs (g)	Total Sugar (g)	Fat/ Sat Fat (g)	Fiber (g)	Ph 1	Ph 2	Ph 3
Fruit butter, apple	1 Tbsp	6	5	0/0	0	A	A	V
Fruit spreads, 100% fruit	1 Tbsp	10	8	0/0	0	A	A	V
Jam or jelly, light	1 Tbsp	8	5	0/0	0	A	A	V
Jam or jelly, regular	1 Tbsp	13	13	0/0	0	A	A	V
Marmalade, orange	1 Tbsp	13	12	0/0	0	A	A	V
Preserves, reduced-sugar	1 Tbsp	9	7	0/0	0	A	A	V
Preserves, regular	1 Tbsp	13	13	0/0	0	A	A	V

OTHER SUGARS

Food	Portion	Total Carbs (g)	Total Sugar (g)	Fat/Sat Fat (g)	Fiber (g)	Ph 1	Ph 2	Ph 3
Fructose	1 Tbsp	10	10	0/0	0	A	V	L
Sucrose	1 Tbsp	10	10	0/0	0	A	V	L

SUGAR SUBSTITUTES

Food	Portion	Total Carbs (g)	Total Sugar (g)	Fat/Sat Fat (g)	Fiber (g)	Ph 1	Ph 2	Ph 3
Equal (aspartame)	1 tsp	3	0	0/0	0	a	a	a
Splenda (sucralose)	1 tsp	1	0	0/0	0	a	a	a
Sprinkle Sweet (saccharin)	1 tsp	1	0	0/0	0	a	a	a
Sugar Twin (saccharin)	1 tsp	0	0	0/0	0	a	a	a
Sweet'N Low (saccharin)	1 tsp	0	0	0/0	0	a	a	a
Sweet One (acesulfame K)	1 tsp	1	0	0/0	0	a	a	a
Sweet-Ten (saccharin)	1 tsp	0	0	0/0	0	a	a	a

SYRUPS

Food	Portion	Total Carbs (g)	Total Sugar (g)	Fat/Sat Fat (g)	Fiber (g)	Ph 1	Ph 2	Ph 3
Corn syrup, high-fructose	1 tsp	5	5	0/0	0	A	A	A
Honey, commercial blend	1 tsp	6	6	0/0	0	A	A	A
Honey, pure	1 tsp	6	6	0/0	0	A	V	L
Maple syrup, pure	1 tsp	4	4	0/0	0	A	V	L

Food	Portion	Total Carbs (g)	Total Sugar (g)	Fat/ Sat Fat (g)	Fiber (g)	Ph 1	Ph 2	Ph 3
Pancake syrup, imitation, maple	1 tsp	5	4	0/0	0	A	V	L
Pancake syrup, imitation, reduced-calorie	1 tsp	2	2	0/0	0	A	V	L

VEGETABLES

Eat and enjoy plenty of vegetables. They are low in calories but high in vitamins, essential nutrients, and fiber. Look for brightly colored vegetables, which contain antioxidants, such as Vitamins A, C, and E. Opt for as much variety as possible, and yes, even carrots are fine. In addition to their nutrient contribution, vegetables, especially when eaten raw, are a great source of fiber and bulk. When cooked in water, vegetables quickly lose their nutrients, so when you cook your vegetables do so in as little water as possible, and for as short a time as possible.

Food	Portion	Total Carbs (g)	Total Sugar (g)	Fat/ Sat Fat (g)	Fiber (g)	Ph 1	Ph 2	Ph 3
Artichokes	½ cup	8	1	0/0	4	G	G	G
Asparagus	½ cup	2	0	0/0	1	G	G	G
Beans, green	½ cup	4	1	0/0	2	G	G	G
Beets	½ cup	8	6	0/0	1	A	V	V
Bok choy	½ cup	2	0	0/0	0	G	G	G
Broad beans (fava)	½ cup	8	1	0/0	2	L	L	G
Broccoli	½ cup	4	2	0/0	2	G	G	G
Broccoli rabe	½ cup	3	1	0/0	0	G	G	G
Brussels sprouts	½ cup	4	1	0/0	2	G	G	G
Cabbage, green or red	½ cup	2	1	0/0	0	G	G	G
Carrots	½ cup	6	2	0/0	2	A	G	G

VEGETABLES (CONT.)

Food	Portion	Total Carbs (g)	Total Sugar (g)	Fat/ Sat Fat (g)	Fiber (g)	Ph 1	Ph 2	Ph 3
Cauliflower	½ cup	3	1	0/0	1	G	G	G
Capers	1 Tbsp	0	0	0/0	0	G	G	G
Celeriac	½ cup	7	1	0/0	1	G	G	G
Celery	½ cup	2	1	0/0	0	G	G	G
Chayote squash	½ cup	3	1	0/0	1	G	G	G
Chicory, raw	1 cup	4	0	0/0	3	G	G	G
Chives, raw	2 Tbsp	0	0	0/0	0	G	G	G
Cilantro, raw	2 Tbsp	0	0	0/0	0	G	G	G
Collards	½ cup	1	0	0/0	0	G	G	G
Corn, sweet	½ cup	15	2	1/0	2	A	V	V
Cucumber, raw	½ cup	1	0	0/0	0	G	G	G
Daikon radish, white	½ cup	2	1	0/0	0	G	G	G
Dandelion greens, raw	1 cup	3	1	0/0	0	G	G	G
Eggplant	½ cup	2	1	0/0	1	G	G	G
Endive, raw	1 cup	2	0	0/0	2	G	G	G
Fennel	½ cup	3	0	0/0	1	G	G	G
Garlic	1 clove	1	0	0/0	0	G	G	G
Ginger, juice or grated	1 tsp	0	0	0/0	0	G	G	G
Green onion (scallion), raw	2 Tbsp	1	0	0/0	0	G	G	G
Hearts of Palm	½ cup	2	0	0/0	0	G	G	G
Kale	½ cup	3	1	0/0	0	G	G	G
Jicama	½ cup	6	1	0/0	3	G	G	G
Kohlrabi	½ cup	4	2	0/0	2	G	G	G
Leeks	½ cup	6	2	0/0	0	G	G	G

Food	Portion	Total Carbs (g)	Total Sugar (g)	Fat/ Sat Fat (g)	Fiber (g)	Ph 1	Ph 2	Ph 3
Lettuce, raw	1 cup	1	0	0/0	0	G	G	G
Mushrooms	½ cup	4	0	0/0	0	G	G	G
Mustard greens	½ cup	1	0	0/0	0	G	G	G
Okra	½ cup	4	1	0/0	2	G	G	G
Onions	½ cup	9	3	0/0	1	G	G	G
Parsley, raw	2 Tbsp	0	0	0/0	0	G	G	G
Parsnips	½ cup	12	3	0/0	3	V	V	L
Peas								
Green	½ cup	10	4	0/0	4	A	G	G
Snow, pod	½ cup	5	3	0/0	1	G	G	G
Sugar snap	½ cup	8	4	0/0	2	G	G	G
Pepper, bell, yellow, orange, red or green	½ cup	3	2	0/0	1	G	G	G
Pepper, chile, raw	2 Tbsp	2	1	0/0	0	G	G	G
Potatoes, baked, w/skin								
Extra-large	12 oz	86	5	0/0	8	A	A	V
Large	8 oz	57	4	0/0	5	A	A	V
Medium	5 oz	36	2	0/0	3	A	A	V
Small	3 oz	21	1	0/0	2	A	A	V
Potatoes, other								
Instant mashed (prepared)	½ cup	11	1	5/3	0	A	A	V
Mashed, regular, plain, no fat	½ cup	15	1	0/0	3	A	A	V
Microwaved, whole	5 oz	34	2	0/0	3	A	A	V
New, whole	2½ oz (3 each)	9	0	0/0	1	A	V	V

VEGETABLES (CONT.)

Food	Portion	Total Carbs (g)	Total Sugar (g)	Fat/ Sat Fat (g)	Fiber (g)	Ph 1	Ph 2	Ph 3
Pumpkin	½ cup	4	4	0/0	0	A	L	L
Purslane	½ cup	1	0	0/0	0	G	G	G
Radish, red	½ cup	2	1	0/0	0	G	G	G
Rutabaga	½ cup	6	4	0/0	2	A	L	L
Sauerkraut	½ cup	3	1	0/0	2	G	G	G
Seaweed, dried	1 oz.	23	0	0/0	2	G	G	G
Shallots	2 Tbsp	3	1	0/0	0	G	G	G
Sorrel, raw	2 Tbsp	1	0	0/0	0	G	G	G
Spinach, raw	1 cup	1	0	0/0	0	G	G	G
Sprouts, alfalfa, raw	½ cup	1	0	0/0	0	G	G	G
Squash, yellow summer	½ cup	2	1	0/0	0	G	G	G
Squash, spaghetti	½ cup	3	0	0/0	½	G	G	G
Sweet potato, cubes, baked	½ cup	21	11	0/0	2	A	G	G
Swiss chard	½ cup	1	0	0/0	0	G	G	G
Tomato, ripe	1 cup	8	5	½/0	2	G	G	G
Tomatoes, cooked	½ cup	5	3	0/0	0	G	G	G
Tomatillo, raw	1 cup	8	3	1½/0	3	G	G	G
Turnip Greens	1 cup	4	0	0/0	2	G	G	G
Turnip	½ cup	4	2	0/0	1	A	G	G
Watercress	½ cup	0	0	0/0	0	G	G	G
Water chestnuts	½ cup	15	3	0/0	2	G	G	G
Wax beans	½ cup	4	2	0/0	2	G	G	G
Yam, cubes, baked	½ cup	19	1	0/0	3	A	G	G
Zucchini	½ cup	2	1	0/0	0	G	G	G

THE SOUTH BEACH SUPERMARKET CHEAT SHEET

There's nothing worse than arriving home from work hungry and discovering that the cupboard is bare. Keep the following staple items in your freezer and pantry, and you'll always have the makings of a healthy South Beach meal.

Dairy

Reduced-fat or fat-free cheese: Try American, Cheddar, mozzarella, ricotta, and Swiss—you'll find countless varieties. Experiment with different brands until you find one you like.

Fat-free plain yogurt: Use it as a staple for making "cream" sauces or dips. (Put it in a sieve lined with a coffee filter and refrigerate it for 3 or more hours, then combine it with your favorite seasonings.)

Flavor Boosters

Balsamic vinegar: It wakes up salads, is a fat-free way to sauté, and is great combined with olive oil in marinades.

Garlic: No well-stocked kitchen is complete without garlic, a staple of Mediterranean cuisine.

Olive and canola oils. For the best-tasting salad dressings, light sautéing, dips for bread, or dressing for steamed vegetables, buy extra virgin olive oil. Canola oil is good for stir-fries.

Onions: Keep a couple of these on hand: red, yellow, and white onions; shallots; and scallions.

Salsa: Use fresh or jarred salsa in place of ketchup and as an accompaniment for grilled meat, poultry, or seafood.

Sesame oil and reduced-sodium soy sauce: These flavor boosters add instant Asian flavor to steamed vegetables, stir-fries, and marinades. Refrigerating these items will help them preserve their flavor if you don't use them up quickly.

Meat, Poultry, and Fish

Boneless top sirloin: For quick and easy beef-and-vegetable kebabs, skewer the meat with mushrooms and chunks of red pepper and onion.

Boneless turkey and chicken breast: Grill it, bake it, or use it in stir-fries.

Veggies and Beans

Beans: Try all kinds—black, butter, lentils, limas, kidney, chickpeas, green, Italian, and split peas.

Frozen vegetables: Keep broccoli and cauliflower florets, asparagus, and chopped spinach on hand for stir-fries, sautéed or microwaved side dishes, additions to casseroles and soups, and Mediterranean dishes like ratatouille.

Prewashed, prepackaged broccoli florets: Serve them as no-fuss crudités with reduced-fat or fat-free cheese, sauté them with black beans as a side dish, or add them to a ready-made soup.

MEDLEY OF MENU MAKEOVERS

It's one thing to follow a straight-from-the-book diet plan, quite another to assemble your own healthy meals. But it's not as hard as it may seem. Simply pair a serving of lean protein with a serving of fiber-rich, fresh veggies (other than high-glycemic varieties like corn and potatoes). Add a dash of healthy oils. Presto—you've got a delicious meal that slows your digestion and keeps you feeling satisfied for hours.

These before-and-after breakfast, lunch, and dinner "makeovers" will help inspire you to think of your own tempting combos. Pair what you know about the nutritional principles of the diet with your own favorite foods and a little creativity and the sky's the limit.

SWITCH FROM THIS . . .	. . . TO THIS

BREAKFAST

Omelet with cheese, hash browns, bacon or pork sausage, and orange juice (from concentrate)	Veggie omelet, Canadian bacon, an orange, and fat-free milk
Plain bagel and a mocha latte	One slice whole wheat toast with no sugar-added peanut butter and coffee with 1% milk and sugar substitute
Pancakes topped with syrup	Whole grain pancakes topped with fresh fruit

LUNCH

Salad with fat-free dressing and pasta with red sauce	Tossed salad with olive oil and vinegar dressing (vinaigrette) and whole grain pasta with shrimp and veggies
Cheeseburger and fries	Grilled chicken breast sandwich on a whole grain roll
Veggie wrap	Tuna salad and veggies wrapped in lettuce

DINNER

Fried chicken, white rice, and a biscuit	Baked chicken breast, steamed asparagus, and a tossed salad with vinaigrette
Meat loaf, mashed potatoes, and bread spread with margarine	Broiled sirloin steak, sweet potato, and oven-roasted veggies
Pork barbecue on a bun, corn, and a tossed salad with fat-free dressing	Cup of tomato soup, open-faced roast beef sandwich, and a tossed salad with vinaigrette

THE SOUTH BEACH
DINING-OUT GUIDE

You don't have to stop frequenting your favorite restaurants just because you're on the South Beach Diet. This way of eating is flexible so that you can find several healthy choices that allow you to enjoy the dining-out experience and still lose or maintain weight. This cheat sheet will help you select the healthiest choices virtually anywhere—even at ethnic restaurants.

Regardless of which Phase of the Diet you're on, be guided by the ground rules for South Beach eating.

Chain Restaurants

Upscale chains offer so much variety that there's plenty to choose from other than deep-fried appetizers, huge entrée portions, and frozen margaritas. At all chain restaurants, avoid appetizers smothered in cheese and sour cream (such as nachos or potato skins), sandwiches called melts (tuna melt, for instance, which are loaded with cheese and grilled with butter), croissant sandwiches, coleslaw, macaroni and potato salads, and fried tortilla shell or bread "bowls."

Try these instead:

At Boston Market: A quarter of a chicken, white meat, no skin or wing; a chicken, turkey, or ham sandwich without cheese or dressing; any fresh vegetable, such as green beans or broccoli.

At Chili's: The Guiltless Grill items, which are usually served with black beans or steamed veggies; shrimp, chicken, or beef fajitas, topped with salsa and minus the flour tortillas and full-fat cheese and sour cream.

At Ruby Tuesday: The salad bar, which contains all the makings for a healthy salad (greens, chickpeas, fresh vegetables, diced turkey or ham, olive oil and balsamic dressing); a turkey burger without the bun; grilled chicken or grilled-chicken salads without the cheese or deep-fried tortilla bowl.

Chinese Food

To give Americanized Chinese food a South Beach makeover, minimize the huge amounts of saturated fat used to prepare it. Ask that your dish be prepared without MSG, the flavoring agent often used in Chinese cuisine. While it's made from beets, a healthy vegetable, MSG has a very high glycemic index (GI). Try egg drop soup or any combination of steamed fresh vegetables prepared with small amounts of meat, poultry, or seafood. Stay away from: steamed rice (it has a high GI); the deep-fried, crispy noodles; egg rolls; fried dumplings; spareribs; lo mein; moo goo gai pan; Peking duck; and entrées described on the menu as "crispy" or "sweet and sour." Also, many sauces may be thickened with cornstarch. Ask the waiter for sauces prepared without added cornstarch.

Indian Food

Indian food is based on good carbs, particularly legumes like chickpeas and lentils, and veggies such as spinach and eggplant. The downside is its abundance of starchy carbs (like potatoes) and bad fats. Many appetizers are deep-fried, and vegetables and meats are typically fried or sautéed in the Indian butter called *ghee*. Still, most Indian restaurants provide several tasty choices for the South Beach dieter. Try Mulligatawny soup, dals (legume dishes—choose those without cream), chana (chickpea curry), kachumbars (vegetable salads), raitas (salads with a tart yogurt dressing), or dishes described on the menu as masala (a combination of spices with sautéed tomatoes and onions) or tandoori (seasoned meat, poultry, or fish roasted in a clay oven).

Stay away from Samosas (deep-fried pastry filled with vegetables or meat); puri (a puffy, deep-fried bread); and entrées described as biryani, malai, or korma, which are heavy on the oil and cream.

Italian Food

Not order pasta? At an Italian restaurant? Actually, it's easier than you think—there are usually several choices right for the South Beach dieter. Try salads dressed with oil and balsamic vinegar; clams steamed in white wine; clear soups; grilled meat, poultry, or fish; scallops sautéed with mushrooms and marsala wine sauce; or escarole or broccoli rabe (two types of greens) sautéed in garlic and olive oil.

If you order pizza, request a thin-crust pie rather than Sicilian or deep-dish, and pile it with veggies rather than sausage or pepperoni. If you must have pasta, ask for whole wheat pasta and order a side serving sautéed in olive oil and garlic or topped with plain tomato sauce and good proteins (clams or shrimp) or vegetables. Stay away from bread or garlic bread; antipastos with cheeses and salami, which are high in saturated fat; and anything described on the menu as "carbonara" (prepared with full-fat cream and cheese) or parmigiana (breaded, fried, and smothered in full-fat mozzarella).

Mexican Food

Most Mexican food at chain restaurants and Mexican fast-food places is prepared American-style, which means an abundance of bad fats. Yet it is possible to go Mexican and eat healthfully. Try grilled chicken or fish, *pescado Veracruzana* (fish in a tangy sauce of olive oil, grilled onions, green olives, and capers), *mole pollo* (boned chicken breast served in a hot and spicy sauce), *mojo pollo* (chicken in a tangy citrus sauce), or *camarones de hacha* (shrimp sautéed in a red and green tomato sauce). Stay away from deep-fried tortilla chips; anything topped with cheese, sour cream, or guacamole; refried beans (commonly fried in lard); chimichangas (deep-fried flour tortillas filled with meat and cheese); the Mexican sausage called chorizo; and deep-fried taco-shell bowls.

Steak Houses

You should be able to have a good South Beach meal in a restaurant specializing in steaks and vegetables. Order a lean cut of meat and enjoy it with a cup of broth-based soup and a side dish of steamed or grilled vegetables.

Try lean cuts of beef such as top sirloin or tenderloin or a well-trimmed lamb or pork loin chop (ask that the extra fat be trimmed away before cooking). At the salad bar, opt for peel-and-eat shrimp, shrimp cocktail, and salad greens with broccoli and other nonstarchy vegetables dressed with olive oil and balsamic vinegar.

Stay away from deep-fried appetizers, creamy soups such as New England clam chowder, baby back ribs, coleslaw, macaroni and potato salads, baked potatoes, steak fries, and onion rings.

S ince the diet became popular in Miami and the book *The South Beach Diet* became a bestseller, I've heard from countless people eager to tell me about their weight loss successes. I'm encouraged by how easy the program is to learn and put into practice. Now there is a Web site designed to make the diet even easier: www.southbeachdiet.com/rodale.

How? The Web site has the flexibility to provide personal feedback and guidance to help you reach your goals. It also has the ability to put you in touch with thousands of others following the plan. In the Message Boards, you'll be able to ask questions and get answers from a large community of dieters with similar experiences, as well as from our expert nutritionists. You'll get regular advice from me, too, in the Daily Dish newsletter and the Ask Dr. Agatston Q&As.

The site's interactive tools are also designed to provide personal support. In the Weight Tracker, for instance, you can key in your weight, chart your progress, and get immediate feedback on how you're doing on the diet. The site will tell you if you're losing weight too fast or too slow, and what you can do about it. It's like having your own personal trainer pointing out areas for improvement, telling you that you're doing better than you think, and keeping you motivated.

In the Meal Plans section of the site, you'll find Daily Menus for whatever phase of the diet you're in, a Recipe Search to help you find delicious new dishes quickly and easily (including vegetarian-only recipes), and a Shopping List Generator that will print out lists of ingredients automatically. By following the South Beach Diet Online, you'll not only get help gaining control of your weight and your heart health, you'll also be helping us make the diet better. Science is changing and improving all the time, and I see this diet as an evolution. As we learn new information about dieters' needs and experiences, we'll be able to continually improve the Web site, the plan, and our ability to help people. To learn about changes and updates to the diet without registering for this site, visit www.southbeachdiet.com/updates.

Arthur Agatston, M.D.

INDEX

Underscored page references indicate boxed text.

A

Alcohol, 13, 19, 21, 27, 40–41
Animal fats, 79

B

Bacon, 101
Bagels, 45
Bars
    breakfast, 48–49
    candy, 55–57
    cereal, 48–49
    meal replacement, 95–96
Beans, 37–39, 129, 135
Beef, 16, 18, 97–99, 134
Beer, 19, 40
Beverages, 24, 40–45, 89. *See also
    specific types*
Bread and bread products, 5, 21,
    27, 45–48. *See also specific
    types*
Bread crumbs, 47
Breadsticks, 47
Bread stuffing, 47
Breakfast bars, 48–49
Breakfast foods, 5, 22, 48–55. *See
    also specific types*
Breakfast makeover, 137
Briskets, 98
Broccoli, 135
Buns, 47–48, 53–54
Burgers, 73–76, 104
Butter, 78–79
Buttermilk, 107

C

Cakes, 65–66
Candy, 5, 55–57
Cane sugar, 127
Canned food, 85, 86–87, 108
Capon, 121
Cappuccino, 42
Carbohydrates, 1, 3, 8–9, 12–13, 19,
    32–33
Carbonated drinks, 41–42
Cereals, 49–51
Cereal toppings, 51–52
Chain restaurants, 138–39
Cheat sheet for South Beach Diet,
    133–35
Cheese and cheese products, 16–17,
    18, 57–60, 133. *See also
    specific types*
Cheese substitutes, 60
Chicken, 76–77, 116–19, 134
Chinese food, 139
Chocolate, 21. *See also* Candy
Chocolate milk, 107
Cholesterol, 11
Clams, 85
Coffee, 42
Condiments, 61, 80–81
Cookies, 66–67
Cornish hen, 121
Cottage cheese, 58
Cow's milk, 107
Crab, 85
Crackers, 62
Cravings, 27–28

Crayfish, 86
Cream, 104–5
Cream cheese, 58, 60
Creamers, nondairy, 105
Croissants, 54
Croutons, 47
Cured pork, 101

D

Dairy drinks and mixes, 43
Dairy products. *See specific types*
Desserts, 5–6, 21, 41, 65–69,
    92–94
Dining-out guide, 138–42
Dinner makeover, 137
Dips, 6, 63
Doughnuts, 54
Dry milk, 108
Duck, 121

E

Eggnog, 107
Eggs and egg dishes, 17, 22, 70–73
Egg substitutes, 73
Espresso, 42
Exercise, 30

F

Fast food, 6, 52, 73–77
Fats, 1–3, 4–7, 17, 33–34, 78–81. *See
    also specific types*
Fava beans, 129
Fiber, 34–35
Fish, 16, 82–85, 133
Flavor boosters, 17, 134
Food guide, using, 31–36
Frozen foods, 7, 93–94, 135
Fruits, 19, 20, 20–21, 86–89, 127

G

Gelatin, 67
GI, 14–15, 139
GL, 15
Glucose, 14–15
Glycemic index (GI), 14–15, 139
Glycemic load (GL), 15
Goose, 121
Grains, 90–91
Gravies, 91
Ground beef, 99

H

Ham, 101
Headaches, 25
Health benefits of South Beach
    Diet, 10–11
Honey, 21, 33
Hot dogs, 102, 104
Hydrogenated oil, 4

I

Ice cream, 19, 21, 92–93
Indian food, 140
Insulin, 9, 12–13
Insulin resistance, 12–13
Italian food, 140–41

J

Jams, 21, 127
Jellies, 127
Juice-flavored drinks, 43–44
Juices, unsweetened, 89

K

Kefir, 107–8

L

Lamb, 99
Lard, 79
Legumes, 17, 20
Lentils, 37–39
Liquors, 40
Lobster, 86
Low-lactose milk, 107
Lunch makeover, 137
Lunchmeat, 16, 102–3

M

Margarine, 79–80
Marmalades, 127
Mayonnaise, 80
Meal planning, 32
Meal replacement bars and shakes, 95–97
Meats, 16, 97–103, 134. *See also specific types*
Meat substitutes, 104
Menu makeovers, 136–37
Mexican food, 141–42
Milk and milk products, 7, 16, 19, 44, 105–9. *See also specific types*
Miracle Whip-type salad, dressing, 81
Mixed drinks, 40
Monosaturated fats, 2
Mousses, 69
MSG, 139
Muffins, 54
Mussels, 86

N

Nursing mothers, 26
Nut butters, 111
Nuts, 17, 23, 110–11

O

Oils, 7, 81–82
Omega-3 fatty acids, 2–3, 29–30
Omelets, 71–72
Oysters, 86

P

Pancakes, 53
Pasta and pasta dishes, 112–13
Pastries, 54–55
Peas, 37
Peppers, 114
Phase 1 of South Beach Diet, 13, 16–19, 22–25
Phase 2 of South Beach Diet, 13, 20–21, 26–29
Phase 3 of South Beach Diet, 13–14, 28–29
Pickles, 114
Pies, 68
Pizza, 114–16
Polyunsaturated fat, 2, 29–30
Popcorn, 64
Pork, 16, 18, 100–101
Portion size, 32
Potato chips, 64
Potato items, fast food, 77
Poultry, 16, 18, 116–19, 134
Pre-diabetes, 12–13
Preserves, 127
Pretzels, 64

Processed foods, 51, 102–3
Puddings, 21, 68–69

R

Relish, 114
Ribs, pork, 101
Rice, 90–91
Rice cakes, 64
Rolls, 47–48, 54–55

S

Salad dressings, 7, 123–24
Salads, 7, 121–23
Sandwiches, 52, 73–76, 102–3
Saturated fats, 3
Sauces, 92
Sausages, 103
Scallops, 86
Scones, 54
Seafood. See Fish; Shellfish
Seasonings, 17, 134
Seeds, 111
Shakes, meal replacement, 96–97
Shellfish, 16, 85–86
Shrimp, 86
Snacks, 6, 63–65
Soups, 7, 125–26
Sour cream, 106
Soybeans, 39
Soy cheese and cream cheese, 60
Soy milk, 19, 44, 109
Spices, 17, 134
Spreads, 79–81, 111
Sprouts, bean, 39
Starches, 19, 20, 21
Steak houses, 142
Steaks, beef, 98
Stews, 7

Sugar, 9, 12–13, 33, 128
Sugar alcohols, 24–25
Sweeteners and sweet substitutes,
    127–29
Sweets, 18. See also Candy; Desserts
Syrups, 33, 128–29

T

Taco shells, 48
Tea, 44
Tempeh, 104
Toaster pastry, 55
Tofu, 17, 104
Toppings, 51–52, 106
Tortillas, 48
Trans fats, 3, 4–7
Triglycerides, 11
Turkey, 119–20, 134

V

Veal, 16, 18, 101–2
Vegetables, 17, 19, 20, 21, 129–32,
    135. See also specific types
Vegetable shortening, 81

W

Waffles, 53
Web site for South Beach Diet, 143
Weight gain, 29
Weight loss, 10–11, 26–27
Whipping cream, 106
Wines, 19, 21, 41
Wraps, fast food, 73–76

Y

Yogurt, 16, 19, 94, 109–10, 133

NOTES

NOTES

NOTES

NOTES

A BESTSELLING PHENOMENON that's **"CHANGING THE WAY AMERICA EATS"**™

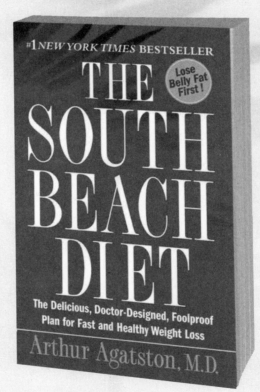

Finally Available in Paperback!

≈ St. Martin's Press